ASTROLOGY OF

INTIMACY, SEXUALITY & RELATIONSHIP

"The answer is to learn about love wisely, rather than passionately . . . Love must facilitate partnership. Respect of individualism between two people looking in the same direction will allow intimacy when the mutual respect pushes criticism away. Personal shortcomings are not ignored, rather, they become part of the realistically bound profiles.. . . .

"In this process, complementarity (led by astrological need and gain) builds strength. Synastry shows togetherness and teamwork. Love is comfort rather than burden."

—Noel Tyl

An Exceptionally Insightful Guide to Relationship Analysis

Master astrologer Noel Tyl presents the definitive guide to astrological understanding of intimate relationships. Written for intermediate-to-advanced level astrologers, this book provides practical and proven instruction in counseling techniques. Also included are fascinating case studies, along with in-depth analysis of the following relationship aspects revealed in the horoscope:

- Individual behaviors and the prescriptions of the environment
- Intimacy needs revealed in synastry
- Expressions of the Animus and Anima
- Fear and disillusionment
- Fateful connections through the Nodes
- Sexuality: its problems, passions, and extremes
- Moon-Marriage orientation
- Happy relationships; Problem measurements

About Noel Tyl

Noel Tyl is one of the foremost astrologers in the world. His twenty-nine textbooks have led the teaching of astrologers for two generations. Tyl has written the professional manual for the field, the 1,000-page text *Synthesis & Counseling in Astrology*, that has securely placed astrology in company with the most sophisticated disciplines of humanistic studies extant today; most recently, *Astrological Timing of Critical Illness*, which establishes a breakthrough position between astrology and medical diagnosis; and *The Creative Astrologer*, a master treatise on creative and concise techniques of counseling.

Tyl is a graduate of Harvard University in Social Relations (Psychology, Sociology, and Anthropology). He lectures constantly in seventeen countries, and maintains a client list of individuals and corporations throughout the world. His office and home are in the Phoenix, Arizona, area in the United States.

To Write to the Author

If you wish to contact the author or would like more information about this book, please write to the author in care of Llewellyn Worldwide and we will forward your request. Both the author and publisher appreciate hearing from you and learning of your enjoyment of this book and how it has helped you. Llewellyn Worldwide cannot guarantee that every letter written to the author can be answered, but all will be forwarded. Please write to:

Noel Tyl
℅ Llewellyn Worldwide
P.O. Box 64383, Dept. 0-7387-0113-0
St. Paul, MN 55164-0383, U.S.A.

Please enclose a self-addressed stamped envelope for reply, or $1.00 to cover costs.
If outside U.S.A., enclose international postal reply coupon.

Many of Llewellyn's authors have websites with additional information and resources. For more information, please visit our website at www.llewellyn.com.

ASTROLOGY OF INTIMACY, SEXUALITY & RELATIONSHIP

INSIGHTS TO WHOLENESS

NOEL TYL

2002
Llewellyn Publications
St. Paul, Minnesota, 55164-0383 U.S.A.

FIRST EDITION
First Printing, 2002

Book design and editing by Connie Hill
Cover design by Gavin Dayton Duffy

Library of Congress Cataloging-in-Publication Data
Tyl, Noel
Astrology of intimacy, sexuality & relationship : insights into wholeness / Noel Tyl. — 1st ed.
p. cm.
Includes bibliographical references (p.) and index.
ISBN 0-7387-0113-0
1. Astrology and sex. I. Title: Astrology of intimacy, sexuality, and relationship. II. Title.

BF1729.S4 T95 2002
133.5′83067—dc21 2001050444

Llewellyn Publications
A Division of Llewellyn Worldwide, Ltd.
P.O. Box 64383, Dept. 0-7387-0113-0
St. Paul, MN 55164-0383, U.S.A.
www.llewellyn.com

Printed in the United States of America on recycled paper

One is always in the dark
about one's personality.
One needs others
to get to know oneself.

C. G. Jung

Recent Books by Noel Tyl

Prediction in Astrology (1991)

Synthesis and Counseling in Astrology—The Professional Manual (1994)

Astrology of the Famed (1996)

Predictions for a New Millennium (1997)

Astrological Timing of Critical Illness (1998)

The Creative Astrologer (2000)

Solar Arcs: Astrology's Most Successful Predictive System (2001)

Llewellyn's New World Astrology Series, edited by Noel Tyl

How to Use Vocational Astrology for Success in the Workplace

How to Personalize the Outer Planets: The Astrology of Uranus, Neptune and Pluto

How to Manage the Astrology of Crisis: Resolution Through Astrology

Exploring Consciousness in the Horoscope

Astrology's Special Measurements: How to Expand the Meaning of the Horoscope

Sexuality in the Horoscope

Communicating the Horoscope

Astrology Looks at History

Table of Contents

Appreciation

This book deals with deeply personal dimensions of our developmental process. The overall thesis of our work rests upon and is illuminated by the individual's emergence in the process of becoming, in the complex interaction with others working similarly to reach the Ssun.

Among the twenty-nine cases shared here, you will find the life story told many times in the words of the clients, revealing what they have been able to glean, organize, and learn from the astrological process. This individualizes the astrology directly.

We must give appreciation to all the clients who have graciously allowed their developmental paths to be shared here.

Noel Tyl
Fountain Hills, Arizona
April, 2001

Horoscope Charts

1

INTIMACY

Elusive Grace, Common Fear

There is little doubt that aloneness is hostile to the human condition. In a primal sense, aloneness eliminates our potential for reproduction: alone, we cannot fulfill our instinctive human function to create facsimile; we cannot go forth, be fruitful, and multiply. In short, when we are alone, we do not have our Selves confirmed.

The Yin has no Yang. The Ascendant has no Descendant. One half the horoscope is without the other.

Relationship is what everyone wants—every astrologer, psychotherapist, social scientist, clergyperson knows that. Relationship ranks with money and job success as the top targets of life development, as voiced by clients, patients, students . . . by everyone. Indeed, the role of relationship to confirm Self is not always focused *upon another person:* there is the relationship to God, to an idea, to a memory that can define identity powerfully. Difficulties in interpersonal relationships can drive a person to substitute other interaction; there can be alliance with the ephemeral, the revolutionary, the inspirational . . . and even the fixatedly delusional. The point is that it is the essence of relating to *something* that confirms and justifies existence.

Intimacy—which word is derived from roots meaning *extremely inward, deeply within*—**confirms identity deep inside**, provides reflection of the Self from a significant external source; it embodies the

Libran, Venusian archetype, the balance of one's identity. Intimacy invites in the "significant other," the outer part of personal existence. Intimacy is the other hand that is necessary to create applause, to clap, to make the sound of contact; it is the other hand that is necessary to clasp for strength, to make the bond of togetherness, to leave aloneness behind. Intimacy is our relationship with the nearest representative of the external environment.

Astrologically, the Hermetic philosophy: *As above so below,* is completed through intimacy: the Midheaven-Immum Coeli axis is complemented by the cross-continuum, the Ascendant-Descendant axis, *As within so without.* Both axes together tell us who we are.

Yet, while intimacy is so clearly essential, helpful, safe-making, and fulfilling, it is startlingly elusive to attain. Its grace is very difficult for many of us to find. Surprisingly, it is common for us actually *to fear* intimacy, to fear that which we seek so intently. It is sad that we are taught—and we learn—throughout our lives, from early on especially, all the dangers of being intimate—the fears of getting too close—without our being taught the refining grace within intimacy and how to attract holistic complementation with a significant other.

In the context of this study, this book, our hypothesis is that we do not understand intimacy and why it *is* elusive; we must find out *what* it is, within and for each individual.

We think we understand sex—the second part of this study. Too often, it is a mistaken substitute for that which we think promotes or confirms intimacy. We are so easily victimized by our sexual needs—when intimacy is not there to reassure us, when trust is not there to keep us safe—that we quickly divert or repress those vital energies. We must find out how to live more confidently with the sexual drive and help the people we serve as astrologers to do so as well.

Even if we do not understand the make-up of intimacy, even though we fear being intimate and tend to repress sexual energies, it is still the human condition *to expect fulfilling relationships with all their benefits!* We seek relationships constantly; we assume them as our human right; we pretend about them with all kinds of socially keyed behaviors. And, all too often, in this common disposition, we become more alone than ever.

Early Conditioning and Values

Even before each of us is born, a behavioral role-profile is established for us by society and our family. It prescribes by our gender how we are to behave for our entire life. It is on this role profile that our capacity for intimacy is built.

"The doctor told us that we're going to have a boy!"

"I dreamed so clearly the other night—and (what a coincidence!) my mother did too—that we're going to have a baby girl!"

This knowledge immediately sets into motion a cultural avalanche of role prescription, telling us how we will behave with the child who will be born; an identification process that tells us what is expected of the child, that defines who the child is for all to know. The baby's room, clothing, and toys: blue for the boy, pink for the girl, shorts or dresses, trucks or dolls; the parents' dreams for the child: football player or cheerleader, tycoon or beauty queen—all are set in place and symbolized by the very name that will identify the child for its entire life: Jonathan or Anna, Rocky or Betty Sue, Ivan or Tanya. All in place even *before* we are born!

The cultural base for a male is a base that rewards aggressive behavior, strength and endurance, the absence of tears, being in control, fighting and winning (in sexuality and crime as well). The cultural base for the female rewards compliance and supportiveness, recognizes heightened emotionalism (moodiness as well), and projects family nurturing and much communication. When male and female relate to each other, the male is the leader, the female the follower; the male works hard and pays the family bills; the female aggrandizes the male, sexually in the main, and supports his plans for the family. Historically, the boy-child is preferred.[1]

---

1 The effort to birth a male heir or the battles over one have changed world history on numerous occasions. It is mainly through the male that social progress in status is possible, traditionally.

While these roles have been adjusted somewhat in the last thirty years or so, the stereotypes still exist in our culture and they are conspicuous among adults today who are over forty, who inherited an even more rigid profile from their parents, and *their* parents before that.

Indeed, the expectancy for maleness is focused within astrology's Mars profile, and the expectancy for femininity is focused within the Venus profile.[2] The man is attached to drive, success, and status; the woman is allied with beauty, peace, and popularity. As the child begins to develop, the balance among these traits responds gradually to the individuation process, as we shall see: one boy will grow to be less aggressive than another boy-man; one girl will grow to be less sexually interested and responsive than another woman. The large spectrum of individualized changes in the balance notwithstanding, the man is still *expected to be* in charge and be basically invulnerable; the woman is *expected to be* attentive and basically dependent, subservient.

These stereotypes are so well known and are now so openly discussed (which does *not* dilute their imprint during development) that much cultural humor (insight) has been attached to them. We *know,* for example, that the man driving his family car will *never* stop to ask directions; but the wife is expected to call for help at any time! The damsel in distress gives the man a chance to prove himself and save the day; the man asking for help exposes his vulnerability! This is an echo of the chivalric code, the behavioral prescriptions for knights of yore.

In the early homelife and in school—and in the public media—the little boy or little girl is treated *according to these culturally prescribed behavioral profiles.* The parents' parents taught this practice and lived it. The parents will now continue it and, in the process, become *the founders of our value structure,* that which accompanies us for better or worse into much of our life.

---

2 We can note the runaway best-selling book, presently a television series as well, topping the charts for several years, titled *Men Are from Mars; Women Are from Venus,* by John Gray (HarperCollins, 1992).

Indeed, our developing culture will alter some of the colors and balances of the stereotypes, of our value structure, but the distinctions and thrusts remain identifiably male-female, Mars-Venus. And even more than by teaching these behaviors in the early home, **the parents influence the children mightily by modeling these behaviors themselves.**

The parents will have also grown up fighting the war between cultural behavioral expectation and their individual needs to exhibit certain specific behaviors. The result, the patterning of the behaviors into routine, becomes their identity. **How sensitively and fairly our parents traffic with each other in terms of their individual identity is now put upon their children and displayed to them vividly.**

Ask yourself the following questions:

Did your father ever say, "Doris baby, I love you!" or "Johnny baby, I love you!"? What have you carried forward from that scenario?

How much of the time was your father "there"? Was he active and engaged with your growing up—or only when it suited him? If he was tyrannical, was his behavior with you different than it was with your brothers and/or sisters? How did that make you feel about yourself?

How did your father relate to your mother? What affection did you ever see between them? When you were a teenager, did your parents sleep together in the same bed? What tone did your mother and/or father set when talking with you about sexuality? What values did you walk away with there?

If your mother was "in your way," might she have been acting out onto you her frustrations with her husband? Was that why she competed with you? Was she jealous of her husband's attentions to you, though passive and more pal-like than paternal? Was she running things to justify her marriage decision long before and to emphasize her role-behavior as a woman? Had she subjugated your father into passivity? Why had she needed to do that? Why had he let her? This is an upset of the stereotype role prescriptions in our society; how is that affecting you now in *your* adult relationship?

If your father drank too much, why do you think he did; how might you have been involved? How do you excuse him? If you don't excuse him, what feelings toward him do you still carry with you?

If your mother was sickly much of the time, why do you think that was so? How do you excuse that? How has that role she played touched your life now?

If your mother was the perfect saintly flower, why did she have no say with your father? What skeletons may have been in *their* closets? What may have been unspoken between *them*? How have you brought her bear-it-in-silence poise forward into your life as a woman or a man?

These questions are not surprising questions; they are perfectly routine channels of thought with regard to the roles played out by all parents in our culture, acting out their developmental problems individually and in relation to each other and then patterning their parental behavior for their children. And, no matter how dreadful it was—or, some may say, *because* it *was* so dreadful—**the children very often go on to marry echoes of their parents!** Right now, you can name people whom you know well who have indeed married their father or mother—sometimes several times! This is the developmental phenomenon of getting back to unfinished business, and it is, believe it or not, *how many of us are most comfortable!* We are used to the roles that are being played; and, in that those behaviors are predictable, life is secure; there are no surprises. We act the same way our parents did. We think there is something "right" about that, and we pass it all on to *our* children.

Perhaps your father died or left the family before you could settle things; how do you feel about that? If you idolize your father as the paragon of excellence, are you sure of that image or do you desperately want to see it that way? Maybe you're covering over some dark things with that bright image. You were the "apple of his eye," but what did he do authoritatively to lead you to the best way for you? How do you yourself or your significant other live up to that model in your mind?

Tough questions, for sure, but I have heard many thousands of responses to them over many years, and I know that these questions are not unreasonable. I also know that these questions, discussed with objectivity, knowledge, and grace, can present helpful, liberating answers. They can bring a new, long-overdue focus to personal identity, improving the trust we have in our personal value system or adjusting that value system significantly. This in turn allows us to get closer to the poise that allows intimacy and leads to glowing relationship.

It goes without much reiteration that, as the child works full time to establish a value system to be used to shape thought and guide behavior, *the approval of the father in our society is of prime importance.* The mother has done the birthing; there is a bond there with the child that is primal; *but the relationship with the father is the first foreign one the child has.* The father must be won over to confirm who we are. When these relationships with the mother or the father are out of balance, are bewildering, threatening, or non-existing, the entire developmental system of the child is challenged very strongly.

We shall see shortly that these developmental tensions, these conditions of growing up, are strongly suggested in horoscopes in many ways. Incisive conversation and helpful therapeutic discussion can be initiated very quickly. The astrologer-client relationship then develops strength and significance quickly, through empathy, a very important dimension of intimacy.

Our Individual Needs

As soon as we are born, as we enter into the role-prescription arena, our *individual* development begins as well. Within the set stereotypes, a child with the Moon in Sagittarius, for example, is going to try to develop individualistically differently than the child with the Moon in Capricorn or Scorpio, or Pisces or Cancer. While the child must toe the gender-stereotype line, obey the patterning passed on in one fractured way or another by parents who have already been through it, her/his individual dimensions start to show through, looking for reward, for reinforcement. These individual traits are going to challenge the patterns and the system. *The keenest developmental tension takes place within the interaction between the child's inner environment and his/her external environment.*

From the very first moments of life, parents are constantly looking *for their own traits* within their children. These are the traits that are initially most rewarded with cooing, gurgling, extra bedtime stories, desserts, favoritism in the family, approval of a spouse, money for a new car, inheritance, etc. We children take that parental reinforcement and wear it as a badge of superiority; we base our evaluations, support, and criticism of others upon those reinforced traits. They define us.

This entire, complicated process takes place in the formative early years of our life and is practiced and reinforced further as we children interact with other children. We express ourselves to others as our parents teach us to do, or, in the absence of their involvement, as we are influenced by close friends—usually children with similar problems at home—or by our exposure to the public media, etc. So many problems can enter into this process. These problems undermine self-worth, establish vulnerabilities, and set up fears of personal exposure—all of which work against intimacy, comfortable sexuality, and productive relationships.

John Steinbeck has written, "It is the nature of a man as he grows older . . . to protect against change, particularly change for the better." The social order—as it has been for generations—must be preserved somehow. Society is based upon accumulated samenesses; that is why the Israeli personality, the Egyptian personality, the German stereotype, the Italian, the American are still the same after two hundred or two thousand years.

The prescriptions (the commands, expectations) of the external environment, focused as our super-ego (guiding censorship), are taken on through the parents, the schoolteacher, the boss, the government, the God, driving a hard bargain with emerging individual expression, with any possible divergence from the norm. The external environment may support these attempts for us to be ourselves, reward those attempts, but most often it punishes them to one degree or another. Most often, we are kept in line to be predictable, to be of the mold.

We adjust. Or do we really? Just think of something as out-of-individual-control, as unchangeable as body height. What reward is there for a girl who is "too tall"; or a boy who is "too short"? Think of the years and years and years of looks, mutterings, ostracizing, the pressures for overcompensation, the private times of anguish, all beginning with the parents, implicitly or explicitly, in the home environment establishing the values of our condition!

We can push this further into deeply private issues, if the male sees that his penis is smaller than the norm established through observance of other males; if the female sees herself as conspicuously divergent from the model stereotype of beauty (and/or what her parents expect of her). Self-worth is challenged in development; silent self-deprecation can occur; feelings of inferiority begin; vulnerability is established; the capacity for intimacy is jeopardized; relationships suffer.

Our astrology reflects the beginning of our individuation: it shows us the individual overlay of individualized needs placed upon societal prescription.

The Sun's light energizes our entire system, in the sky and in our being; its light goes everywhere, reflecting to one degree or another on every body in the solar system. The Sun fuels our system. My Capricorn energy, for example, courses through my bodily system and enters into my life, invigorating all my faculties to one degree or another.

The principle focus for the light of the Sun is upon the Moon. Using the Sun's energy, the Moon symbolizes *the reining need of the personality*. There are 144 possible Sun-Moon blends by sign, and these are covered in text images, developed and explored throughout my thousand-page *Synthesis & Counseling in Astrology, The Professional Manual* (Llewellyn, 1994).

The major consideration for us is that *the reigning need of the personality (the Moon), fueled by the energy of the Sun, drives the entire personality to fulfillment.* This individual drive must constantly adapt to societal prescriptions and react to reward and punishments (fulfillment and frustration), beginning with the parents and extending further into the external environment throughout life.

I have the Sun in Capricorn and the Moon in Leo: "In this blend, the energy to organize and deploy resources is 'showcased' for fulfillment: self-dramatization is the mode for persuasion and the call for appreciation. Social evaluation of what one does is taken very personally as evaluation of the personality. The need to be loved is of paramount importance within one's work. Measurements of emotional awareness are necessary elsewhere in the horoscope to soften the picture and help with acceptance." This is basically who I am. Now: how do my faculties for thought, for relating, for energy application, for learning, discipline, dreams, etc. *help me fulfill that primal predisposition?*

Every child's Sun-Moon blend presents a challenge to the parents, which is all the more difficult if the parents have no idea about the astrology of their child. All parents must face how they can support this growth best, wisely, efficiently in their children. **That** is the key. **That** is what is so often not recognized or not respected by the parents (then, extended further: by the spouse, by employers). And this is how fears of criticism, devaluation, and the anxiety about not being understood creep into the personality. Relationships, as we shall see, are the place where these fears are painfully focused. *Intimacy can develop only from personal self-respect and the trust that showing Self to another will not attract criticism, the process of criticism that is most often patterned deeply in the early developmental years.*

In relationship, this inner requirement for us to be ourselves confronts the similar, complicated construct within someone else. The two internal environments try to relate. One must trust the other person in order to be safe, eventually to experience intimacy.

Carrying my personal example further: my father abandoned my mother and me when I was nine. I have no memory of any interaction with him whatsoever before that, or after. My mother seemed to delight in my self-dramatization drive (she had the Sun in Aries, and the Fire-sign affinity with my Leo Moon perhaps helped). And fortunately, when she remarried, my stepfather had no axe to grind, and he delighted in who I was becoming and, more than any soul possibly could, championed and supported that individual growth in me. I was lucky.

The rest of the planets define subsidiary needs: Mercury, how we need to think to be efficient; Venus, how we need to relate; Mars, the kind of energy we need to apply, how we need to apply it, in order to gain fulfillment; Jupiter, the kind of reward that we find most gratifying, the parameters of our learning process; Saturn, our efficiency with the necessary controls we face in the external environment; Uranus, the individuating intensification of who we are; Neptune, the creative visualization process that helps us dream, challenges our perception, and easily touches our faith; and Pluto, the focus of personal empowerment and perspective.

These subsidiary needs, learning faculties, vectors of development come to focus within the wholeness of our personality, serving the reigning need symbolized by the Moon. Planets relate by aspect, and the aspect condition suggests the quality of the interrelationship. Mercury in Capricorn (the need to hear the grass grow, to know detail) is the potential, but when Saturn, as an example, squares it, it will suggest a modification of individual expression, perhaps a somberness or seriousness; Mercury squared by Neptune will take on a different individual expression, etc.

The aspects are like plumbing lines in a twelve-story building: energy is piped from the central source in different ways into different departments of life experience. These departments of life experience are the Houses of the horoscope. And the key Houses in this discussion of individuation and intimacy are the Parental axis (4th and 10th Houses), Self-Worth (the 2nd), and Relationships (the 7th).

We can understand easily that a young boy with the Sun in Cancer, for example, and the Moon in Pisces (the probability of being highly agreeable and pleasant; his personal statement probably diluted by what others want; highly intuitive; a tactful, "sailboat personality"), and perhaps Mars in Pisces as well, may not please his parents easily, *within the stereotype expectations for a boy*. The softer nature of this boy could easily clash with the father's more powerfully anchored persona. The father could easily lose interest, and this child then easily withdraws. How might the child's sensitivity be misinterpreted? What would be the pattern of the parental reaction? Would the mother come to the rescue (the child could have Venus square the Nodal axis)? Would he become a so-called mamma's boy?

What about the young girl whose astrology calls for individuation that is decidedly away from the Venus norm? Would she be labeled "one of the boys," "one of the guys"? How would that fit in where? Would the parents be terribly disappointed in relation to their imaginings for the child even before she was born?[3]

I remember painfully that when my mother and I were living alone for three years or so, she fell and hurt her back severely. I was pushed into doing much housework (my Cancer Ascendant surely opening me to this). She well-meaningly put an apron on me, and I did not mind. I was taking piano lessons and loved it. I was bright and very sensitive. I had no role model as a young male. Although I was much bigger than almost everyone else, I was pudgy and clumsy; I had grown so fast. And then my mother bought me a bicycle—*a girl's bicycle,* probably not knowing any different. I was teased terribly for two years! My middle initial "J" was converted by the other, more masculine boys to "Nole Jane," mispronouncing my first name in the process.

What did that do to me? What *could* that have done to me? Was I self-respecting enough—from my mother's influence and my earliest understandings of who I was—to withstand it?

When my mother remarried—probably in the knick of time—everything changed in what seemed an instant: I very quickly became coordinated and strong, a prominent athlete, my aptitude for music flourished and became a

---

3 I have one female acquaintance who is bright, very musically talented, fun, not unattractive, but very tall, a bit lumbering. Her parents named her "Allan," spelling it in the masculine way (instead of "Allen"). It is astounding how all of this worked together to defeat this woman in her socialization process. She is now coming to the close of her life without ever having had a meaningful relationship with a man.

special reference of achievement—and, yes, I did extract some revenge on those old "friends" (and this delights me still a half-century later!), i.e., with my physical and mental strength I commanded their appreciation of me and I got it.

It is quite sobering and instructive to realize that each person reading these paragraphs has some drama of identity formation to share along these lines. Each of our clients does too.

The points now emerge: how can we trust who we are becoming unless we have *parental involvement and support*? How can we organize the values that guide behavior and feelings without putting *our personal needs and the prescriptions of the environment in good balance*? How strong are we with our sensitivities, our vulnerabilities in life, *to speak of them without fear to someone else, beginning with our parents,* especially the parent of the same gender? **These are the requirements for, the grace of, and the rewards from intimacy;** and this is the magical self-sustaining trust possible in relationship.

Chart 1: "Frances"

This first example horoscope is the first horoscope that came before me on the day I determined the title and path of this book (p. 15). It is a perfect example of all we have discussed so far, and I am very grateful to "Frances" for allowing us to share it.

Orientation outline to the horoscope [presented throughout this book in the style developed strongly in *The Creative Astrologer* (2000)]:

- Western hemisphere emphasis (giving herself away to others; leaving herself behind, perhaps even undeveloped); and to the North (below the horizon), unfinished business in the early homelife.
- Sun-Moon blend in Gemini: energy for brightness, diversification and communication, possible restlessness and indecision; ingenuity and intelligence; needs education for anchor and refinement.
- The Sun-Moon position is a tight New Moon: according to the ancients, usually a difficulty for development, a delayed development,

since the Moon has no light; the wide square to the Sun and the Moon from Saturn in the 7th corroborates this, plays into it, and the observation starts to define a personal vulnerability; Saturn is also tightly square to the Midheaven, one arm of the parental axis; Saturn rules the Ascendant and, in its aspect activity, suggests a depression of identity growth.

- Pluto, ruler of the Midheaven, is (widely) *quindecile* to the Ascendant, suggesting a difficult time developing self-empowerment, perhaps a constant quest to do this.
- Pluto is squared with Mars, co-ruler of the Self-worth 2nd; there is a stress in the self-worth profile; Pluto rules the 9th House as well and, in this tension structure, suggests that the education was interrupted as well.
- The developmental tension is decidedly in the early home environment and *will be played out in relationships:* the Sun and Moon, both squared by Saturn, are co-rulers of the 7th House of relationships.
- Mercury is the final dispositor of the horoscope (in its own sign), is conjoined with Venus (cerebrated idealization, usually an overcompensatory, defensive device) and will be focused strongly within the sex profile since Mercury rules the 5th and the 8th and Venus is co-ruler of the 8th.
- There is an Air Grand Trine (slightly broad, but invited by the client's developmental situation) which is a defensive closed circuit of intellectual and/or social self-sufficiency.
- And finally, there is the important statement of Uranus conjunct the Aries Point promising an unusual individuation finally emerging into the public view (Frances is a talented astrology student) and Mars is oriental, rising last before the Sun does, suggesting a strong promotional ability, a salesmanship, a persuasion, even a teaching modality in expression.

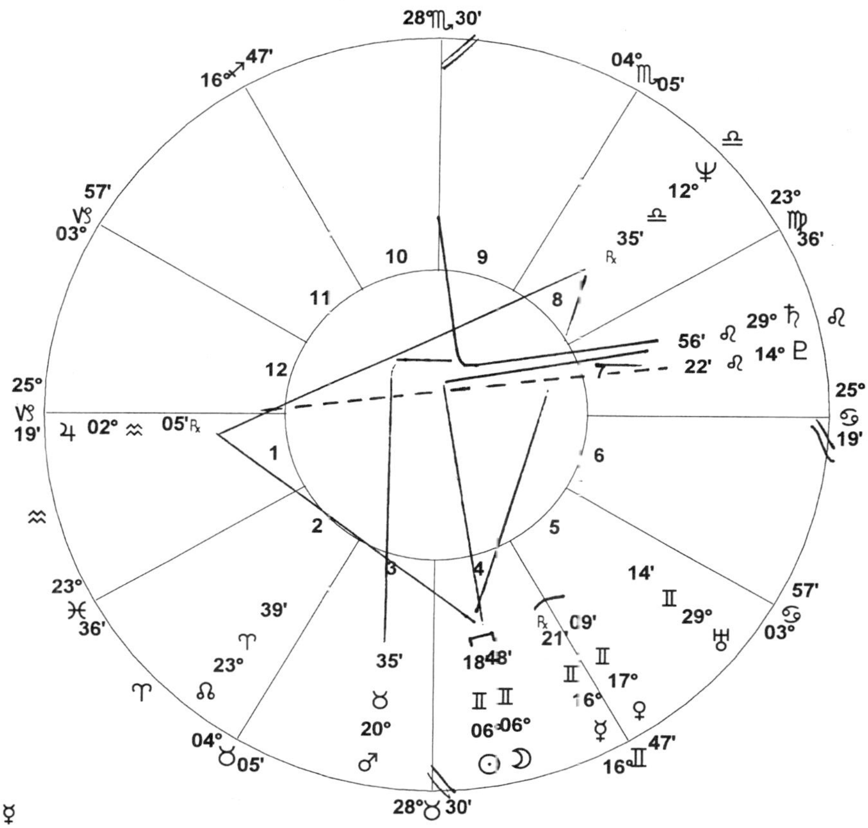

	☽	☉	☿	♀	♂	♃	♄	♅	♆	♇	☊	Mc
☉	☌s 0C°30											
☿		॥										
♀			☌s 00°48									
♂												
♃	△s 04°43	△s 04°13	bQs 00°44	bQs 00°04								
♄	□s 0E°52	□s 06°23	Qs 01°35	Qa 00°46		⊼a 02°10						
♅				॥			⚹a 00°41					
♆	△a 05°47		△a 03°46	△s 04°34			∠s 02°21					
♇	॥		⚹a 01°59	⚹s ॥ 02°47	□			∠a ॥ 00°08	⚹s 01°47			
☊	∠a 01°51	∠a 02°21										
Mc						⚹a ॥ 03°35	□a 01°25	⊼a 00°44	∠s 00°55			
Asc		#			△s 04°43	☌a 06°47			q		□s 01°39	⚹s 03°12

Chart 1

"Frances"

From this outline, it is not difficult to anticipate the developmental scenario in early life, the defensiveness of self-worth vulnerabilities, difficulties in relationship because of the early patterning and accumulated vulnerabilities, and *the keen mind working overtime privately to protect against emotional anxiety with others* [the Air Grand Trine, the loneliness of the New Moon, the retrogradation of Mercury, suggesting a second agenda; the Sun-Moon pipeline into the 7th through the square with Saturn]. The challenge for intimacy is hard for Frances to face.

Now, Frances, with my guidance, had analyzed her horoscope herself and had sent it to me to be checked out. The following are phrases and insights presented *in her words:*

> Energy to communicate with needs to be bright and clever, informed and intense . . . unfinished business in the early homelife . . . restrictions in expressing [myself] caused from early developmental concerns that affect how I relate to others . . . a legacy of inferiority feelings brought on by the father and a potential for a father surrogate in later relationships [to settle the unfinished business].
>
> [There is] social and mental self-sufficiency, a loner here. There is a fear of intimacy because of parental conditioning. Education was interrupted affecting professional development. This in turn affected self-worth, personal and monetary resources and state of mind.
>
> There are suggestions of difficulty in shaping identity, which could result in health problems, mental illness, or self-destructive behavior . . . [I'm] romantically idealistic in giving love and in fantasizing about love.
>
> Self-worth comes from approval of others . . . idealism can run away with or interfere with good financial judgments . . . there is a prominent display of being different, rebellious, intense, inspired, and a love of travel [Uranus conjunct the Aries Point].
>
> I certainly display a lot of antisocial behavior . . . I am very insecure about a lot of things, most importantly, a lack of education, finances, work and relationships. **I need to develop this feeling of security within, and I think this is the key.**

> [In commenting specifically on the Pluto-Ascendant quindecile:] It is suggested that a strong need for personal power and importance is played out through relationships, but it will have difficulty being expressed because of unfinished business in the early home life . . . [therefore] needs are repressed. **Fear of abandonment results in obsessive behavior to control the outcome in relationships.** Oppressive dealings with others create upsets with those in authority. Compulsive behavior towards relationships leads to separation.

I was deeply impressed with the extraordinary honesty of this self-evaluation astrologically. Frances had developed an enriching, objectified view of her development. Now, she could knowingly make adjustments in thought and behavior.

Chart 2: "Ruth"

Chart 2 (p. 19) is "Ruth." Here is a general analytical outline of her horoscope:

- The Sun-Moon blend (Sagittarius-Capricorn) promises assertive opinionation tied with realism, with a helpful dimension of idealism, a worldly sense, that encourages objectivity and compassion at the same time. To thine own self be true.
- The Eastern Hemisphere emphasis of the horoscope suggests a defensive nature. This is magnified by Neptune conjunct the Ascendant opposed by Saturn-retrograde, ruler of the Self-worth 2nd.[4]
- The early home focus is reinforced by Neptune, within the opposition with $Saturn_{Rx}$ and at the Ascendant, ruling the 4th, semisquare the Moon.

---

4 The $Saturn_{Rx}$ phenomenon which I have developed for some thirty years suggests reliably that there is a legacy of inferiority feelings taken on in the early homelife, usually in connection with the father figure in the home, who was either taken out of the picture early, was there and passive, or was so tyrannical—any combination of these—so as never to have given the guidance of authoritative love.

- Pluto opposing Mars in the 4th suggests a battleground in the giving of love (Mars rules the 5th).
- As the complex assembles itself, we must note that Mercury, ruler of the 7th House of relationships, is not under developmental tension *but* the proximity of Saturn$_{Rx}$ to the seventh cusp (arcing there during the formative years of four and five) will probably bring relationships into the quandary of developmental tension.
- Venus in Capricorn almost always carries with it the sense of a delayed emotional development, in this case, the time to work out the problems in the early homelife before being comfortable with giving and receiving love in relationships (Venus rules the 11th, love-received; Mars, opposed by Pluto, rules the 5th, giving love); the sextile between Venus and Mars does not eliminate the difficulties, *but links the concerns for eventual resolution in support (sextile) of the personality.*
- Some dynamic time measures leap out from the natal horoscope: Neptune=Ascendant [Solar Arc Neptune conjoins the Ascendant[5]] at just before three years of age, Saturn=Ascendant just after five years of age; and then the arcs MC=Mars at six, Neptune=Jupiter$_{Asc}$ at sixteen, and Neptune=Sun at twenty-three. These arcs suggest a debilitation (invalidation) even illness (Pluto rules the 12th and is opposed by Mars) for the personality and, curiously, the possible intrusion or rescue by spirituality (Neptune at the Sagittarius ascendant, arcing over Mercury, Jupiter, and the Sun).

In our telephone consultation, Ruth corroborated "precisely" my opening statement about the Sun-Moon blend and the Eastern Hemisphere emphasis. I suggested to her that the short circuit requiring the defensive posture related back to the father and to some very difficult times between the ages of three and five.

---

5 For full presentation of the theory and practice of Solar Arc measurement, prediction past and future, please see Tyl, *Solar Arcs*, Llewellyn, 2001.

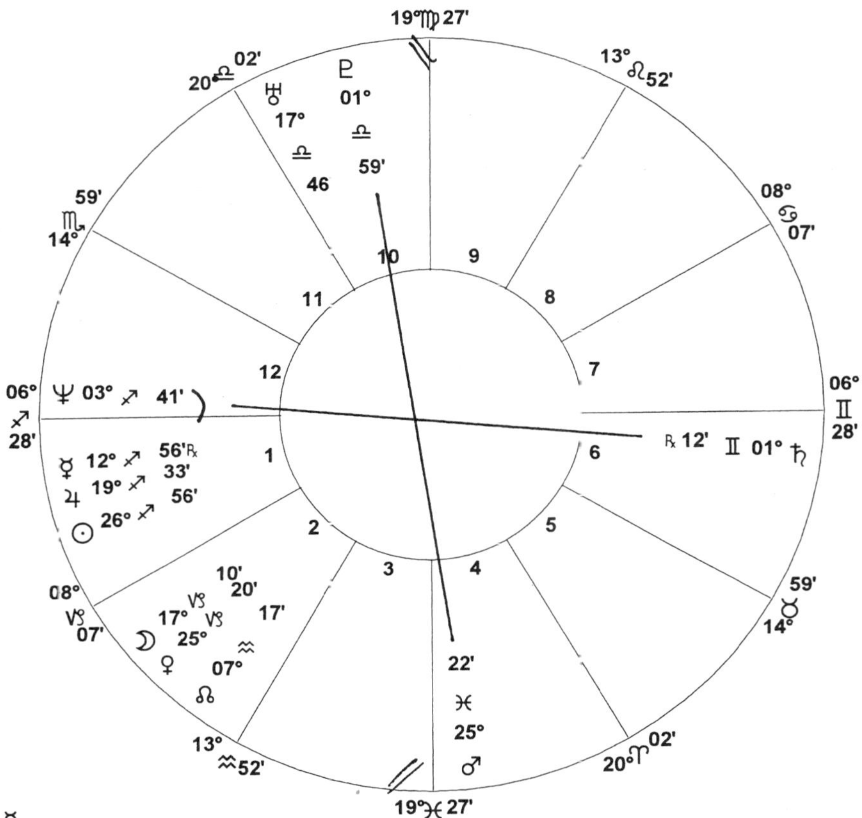

	☽	☉	☿	♀	♂	♃	♄	♅	♆	♇	☊	Mc
☉	∥											
☿												
♀		∥										
♂		□s 01°33		✶a 00°03								
♃		∥	☌s 06°37	∥	□s 05°49							
♄	⚻s 00°59			△a 05°52								
♅	□a 00°35					✶s 01°47	⚻s 01°34					
♆	∠a 01°30		∥				☍s ⋕ 02°29	∠s 00°55				
♇		□a 05°03	Qs 01°02		☍a 06°36		△s 00°47		✶s 01°42			
☊							⋕		✶a ∥ 03°37	△a 05°19		
Mc	△s 02°17			△a 05°53	☍a 05°55	□a 00°06			Qa 02°14			
Asc			☌a 06°28				☍s 05°17		☌s 02°48		✶a 00°49	

Chart 2

"Ruth"

Immediately, Ruth disclosed her condition in development at that time: she was seriously ill with rheumatoid arthritis from ages three to five; braces were put on her legs and ankles. When she was three, her father left the home, abandoning the mother and daughter; he then returned when Ruth was five. These were extremely difficult times for Ruth: she was told that she had a life expectancy of twelve because of her crippling disease, and the father's departure suggested that all really was lost.

When I asked about the *spiritual (!)* dimensions within all of this, Ruth said that they were extreme, that she and her mother were part of a literal religious sect. Ruth went to intense religious schooling in the teachings of that sect, involving male dominance and exorcisms of demons, etc. When the Midheaven arced to opposition with Mars, Ruth was told she was possessed by a demon and that she had to submit to exorcism. Ruth said that, even at so young an age, she disapproved of what was going on and that she consciously played along with the ceremony, making all the appropriate noises and gyrations, just to please everyone.

At age four or five, at a church social gathering, Ruth was touched by a mysterious man who told her that, if she had faith, she would be cured. The next morning she was able to walk; she was cured; and the problems never returned!

Ruth changed schools (tr Uranus conjunct her Ascendant), and at the same time, her father, told that *he* was now demonized, committed suicide.

Clearly, Ruth was developing within a maelstrom of emotions, religious rationale, and the grievous insecurity of father abandonment. Then, the father dimension was compounded dramatically when Ruth was twenty-four [Neptune=Sun, with tr Neptune conjunct Venus and tr Saturn conjunct the fourth cusp]: she was in a relationship, and the man kept information from her until the last minute, that he would leave her and follow his job halfway around the world. Ruth was abandoned yet again.

Ruth shared with me that, in that relationship, she had been all right sexually, "when there *wasn't* a lot of intimacy. He couldn't handle intimacy."

Now, this is a garbled statement: did she do well because he did well, since there was no intimacy demanded from him ("he couldn't handle it")? Or did Ruth do well because she could (had to?) separate sex from intimacy, and therefore avoid exposing her vulnerabilities, *her* fear of abandonment, etc.?

Ruth is now in a super relationship, apparently splendid in every way. "But it has taken us *three years* to get it that way! My problem is my vulnerability, my fear of abandonment . . . the aloneness I fear . . . and I was putting all my father-stuff on him. I was using projection, big time!"

The time needed to solve these problems caused a delay in her emotional maturation (Venus in Capricorn). Ruth worked hard to restore her self-worth by becoming her own boss and building a strong business, through meeting an empathic male who stayed the emotional course of her growth, and through her disarming honesty about herself (astrology study, Buddhism, and more) learning security within her identity.

Ruth is able now to trust herself with her partner, **trust him to care about her weaknesses, fears, and strengths without criticism, rejection, or abandonment.** She can now feel safe. This has restored Ruth almost completely—another cure in her life—and *this intimacy* that has finally arrived has bloomed beautifully within the strengthened relationship.

Chart 3: "Henry"

Chart 3 (p. 23), "Henry," is the client who followed in my schedule right after Ruth. I say this to show that, while these lives disclose dramas that are highly individual, they occur within scenarios of development that are routinely seen. We are guided in each case by astrological dynamics (especially rulership networks among key Houses) and knowledge of the way our family culture raises children. When we are inspecting the tie between developmental tensions in the early home and the adult capacity for and trust of intimacy, we are dealing with a challenge common to us all: very often, analytically, the focus is not whether or not these fears are present *but to what degree they are present*. In each of these cases, we are tracking the links among the 1st, 2nd, 7th, 11th, and 5th Houses in relation to the 4th and 10th. We are seeing early home developmental tensions transferred into self-worth anxiety and relationship difficulty.

The outline of Henry's horoscope [be aware how a creative connectedness is developed throughout the observations]:

- Northern Hemisphere emphasis: unfinished business from the early home.
- Sun-Moon blend: "the energies of uniqueness and the needs to be self-sufficient, right, and in control; the personality feels that it is indispensable. Work with others just proves the fact that the ego is indeed very important."
- Air Grand Trine—closed circuit of social or intellectual self-sufficiency—works to defend against the Saturn retrograde phenomenon; reinforced by Neptune quindecile the Midheaven and Uranus square Venus, ruler of the parental 10th; relationship tensions promised through Uranus rulership of the 7th, sesquiquadrate Mercury ruler of the 11th (love needed, hoped for).
- Moon-Mars opposition on the parental axis; highlighting mother, echoing $\text{Saturn}_{\text{Rx}}$ conjunct the Nodal Axis (the mother runs the show, makes a dominant statement); the Moon is co-ruler of the 11th (a major link here to feelings of not being lovable).
- The midpoint picture Venus=Mercury/Neptune is a very strong statement of romantic idealism, idealization; an echo in the pictures Node=Moon/Venus and Uranus=Node/Asc.
- It is important to note that the Ascendant may be a very powerful "royal" statement here, configured on the ecliptic with the fixed star Regulus.

Henry was twenty-six at the time of our telephone consultation. He did not initially register/recognize any part of the $\text{Saturn}_{\text{Rx}}$ profile. [When this happens, it may be that the client requires time to get underneath the father-*image* to the real role activity within the family, such is the defensive image-

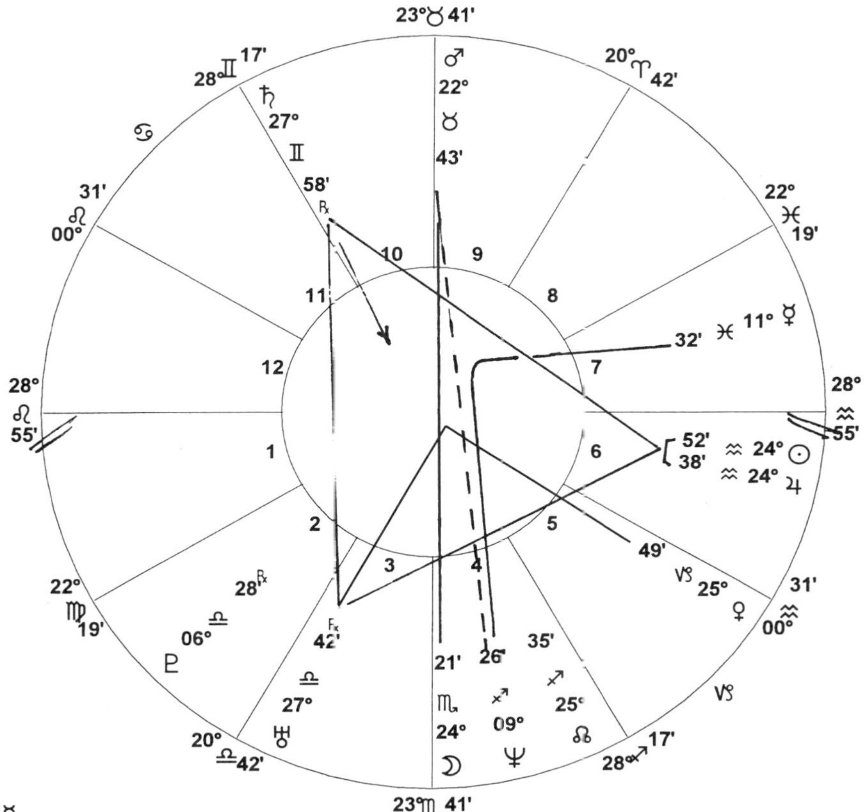

	☽	☉	☿	♀	♂	♃	♄	♅	♆	♇	☊	Mc
☉	□a 00°31											
☿												
♀	⚹a 01°28	ǁ	∠s 00°43									
♂	☍s 01°38	□s 02°09	Qa 00°49	△a 03°06								
♃	□a 00°17	☌s ǁ 00°14		ǁ	□a 01°55							
♄	#	△a 03°06		⚻a 02°09		△a 03°20						
♅		△a 02°50	⚼a 01°10	□a 01°54		△a 03°04	△a 00°16					
♆			□s 02°07	∠s 01°23	q a # 01°42							
♇		#		#	⚼s 01°15	#			⚹s 02°57			
☊		⚹a 00°43				⚹a 00°57	☍s # 02°22	⚹s 02°07				
Mc	☍a 00°40	□a 01°11	Qs 00°09	△a 02°07	☌s 00°58	□a 00°57			q a 00°44	⚼s 02°13	⚻a 01°54	
Asc	□s 04°34	☍s 04°03				☍s 04°17	⚹s 00°57	⚹s 01°13			△s 03°20	□a 05°14

♀ = ☿/♆
alo = ☽/♀
= alo/A

Chart 3

"Henry"

building created by the client to protect or aggrandize the father relationship.] Eventually, Henry was able to describe that his mother *did* "run the show" [a common manifestation of Saturn$_{Rx}$ tightly conjunct or square the Nodal axis]: "And I remember thinking how weak my father was to let this happen."

The mother became a formidable figure in Henry's narrative. Henry then opened up further about his father: "He felt unloved by her [his wife] and was trying to work it out. What *she* loved was the *image* of the family; she had been abandoned by *her* parents."

Henry then said, "*My mother shaped my view of women*, ideally good but also unable to deal with things; [they] can't cope."[6] This is an extremely typical transferal of a parental norm of behavior from the parent to a desired (familiar) state of behavior for the child. This is occurring every time we hear someone say, "I'm really a hard worker like my father; in fact that's what causes . . . ," or "I've inherited this anxiety about my appearance from my mother, for sure; she was always. . . ."

Henry was making references to his emotional relationship difficulties, to women letting him down, confounding his life clearly, *from an identification with his father's perspective, his feelings.*

And, *in the same sentence with his references to his successful job*, Henry juxtaposed mention of relationship difficulties with the evaluation of his job strategies and activities *eighteen times within twenty-minutes minutes!* That is hard to imagine, but it happened during the consultation [I heard it developing and kept score!]. By pointing this out to him, we could see dramatically how success on the job was being complicated by his intensely disruptive relationship life with women and business partners. "Yes, I'm successful in my work, but relationship after relationship broke my heart. My instinct is to love, to empathize, to want intimacy." All of this had driven him into a defensive structure, being separate from the flow, that of an aloof leader.

---

6 When I asked him about ever having seen any intimacy between his father (a doctor) and his mother, he said that he had not.

Henry had been a star: captain of the football team, handsome, talented, creative, had formed his own company, but everything was jumbled up with his enormous need to love and be loved *reliably*. Here again, we can note that Venus is in Capricorn, suggesting a delay in relational value development, in maturation with love matters [Mars square Jupiter, ruler of the 5th; Neptune square Mercury, ruler of the 11th; Mars opposed Moon, co-ruler of the 11th].

Another note is important here: whenever the Sun and Moon are in tight square with each other at birth [the natal chart is a transit chart for the parents], we can reliably surmise that the parents were in conflict when the child was born. Henry's parental situation, though graced with prestige and excellent income, and all the sociometric trappings of a fine family, became heavy emotional baggage for him as a young adult. Understanding this, bringing realistic balance of it all into his life, building his job success *away from an earlier persona* and into a new one was the basis of therapy, helping to free Henry into efficiency with both his worlds.

Chart 4: "Julia"

Our next chart is "Julia's" horoscope (p. 26), showing still another dimension pattern of early home tensions as they build up a fear of intimacy and work against relationship. Here is a brief outline of the horoscope, before we hear the story told in Julia's own words:

- Northwest Hemisphere emphasis: giving one's Self away to others, conditioned by unfinished business in the early home.
- Sun in Libra and the Moon in Cancer: there is an indomitable need here to establish emotional security. The personality is probably flexible and adaptable to the point of self-sacrifice (Western orientation) in order to please others in terms of emotional and home security.
- $Saturn_{Rx}$ phenomenon square $Neptune_{11}$ (and Mars); $Pluto_{7}$ conjoined with $Uranus_{10}$ in the 4th, all suggesting much parental upset that gets played out later in relationships.

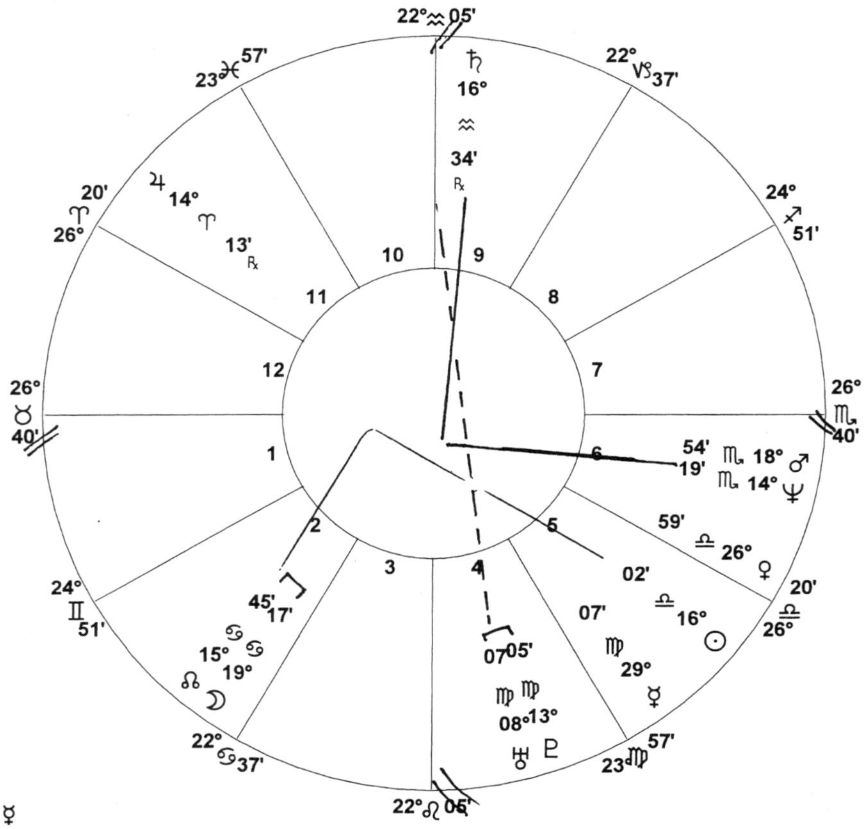

	☽	☉	☿	♀	♂	♃	♄	♅	♆	♇	☊	Mc	
☉	□s 03°15												
☿	Qs 02°10												
♀													
♂	△s 00°22												
♃	□s 05°03	☍s 01°49	q a 00°07										
♄		△a 00°32	⚼a 02°27		□s ‖ 02°21	✶s 02°20							
♅				⫲	Qa 01°13								
♆	△s 04°57		∠a 00°13		☌s 04°35	⊼s 00°06	□a 02°14						
♇				∠a 01°06		⊼a 01°09		☌a 04°57	✶s 01°15				
☊	☌s ‖ 03°32	□s 00°17	Qs 01°21		△s 03°09	□s 01°32	⊼s 00°49		△a 01°26	✶a 02°41			
Mc				△a 04°54	□s 03°10		☌s 05°31	q a 01°03	‖				
Asc			△a 02°26	⊼a 00°18						‖		□a 04°36	Asc

Chart 4

"Julia"

- Uranus quindecile the Midheaven suggests that Julia will find her individuality by obsessively following a work path, a vocational thrust that defines who she is.
- The Sun square with the Nodal axis highlights the mother considerably importantly (in default from SaturnRx); the Sun square with the Moon suggests the parents were already in upheaval at the time of her birth.
- Mercury$_{5,\,2}$ and Venus$_{A,\,6}$, in their own sign, are final dispositors of the horoscope and both are without Ptolemaic aspect, peregrine: an idealistic projection (dissociated somehow, difficult to "plug in"; therefore dominating) of how children or love (5th) should be framed as a personal self-projection, probably the idea of "having it better than I did."

Here are excerpts from a letter Julia wrote to me about her horoscope: "My father, although present with the family, was not emotionally supportive of his family [note the separation; "of us" is clearly avoided] and caused a lot of emotional scarring. All this affects my ability to deal in a healthy 'intimate' relationship."

Julia's father's mother had died when he was two, and he had been raised by a tough father and a disinterested stepmother. Her father had been physically abused throughout his upbringing. Julia sees her father as having the "emotional orientation of a two-year old, seeing the world as totally revolving around him."

With Julia's Sun square the Nodal axis, we can expect a tremendous emphasis on the maternal relationship. Julia's mother made up for everything in the household as supportively as she could.

The parents *were* already in upheaval when Julia was born. [Sun tightly square Moon.]

"I have many male friends, having graduated in Engineering and working in a mostly male field; I tend to feel more at ease with male friendships. I do tend to be very independent, but I believe this to be a mask. The mask is covering my strong fear of intimacy, 'needing to be loved' and feelings of 'I'm not worthy.'"

Note that a peregrine planet can be expected to run away with the horoscope; it searches for "connection" in developmental reality. Here we have a very strong Mercury in Virgo, not only suggesting the mind leading the way in terms of analysis and discrimination, but also bringing far forward self-worth concerns (Mercury rules the 2nd) and the concerns of love and her children (Mercury rules the 5th). Additionally, Neptune, ruling the 11th, is square with Saturn.

Julia's "first love" fathered a child with her, out of wedlock, and abandoned her upon the child's birth. "I realized that all the signs were there of a man who could not meet my very deep emotional needs." [As her father could not.]

"After that relationship, I vowed that I would be very careful not to fall for the same type of man [her Mercury-in-Virgo discrimination strength]." Her next man: "Given all the indications he gave me, I made a conscious decision that this man would be there for my child and me emotionally." [The 5th House prominence in her thinking and feeling; Venus peregrine as well in Libra.]

This man let Julia down by having an affair. Now: "I am questioning my ability to make the right choices. I thought I was aware of why I had chosen to be in the relationship, but I just repeated the pattern!!! Now I am struggling with what is the best situation for my children. I want to break the cycle for their sake. I want to make sure that I provide them with an emotionally healthy environment so that they can grow up knowing what that feels like and recognizing when things are not right.

"I have learned that, while I am working on 'my stuff,' the other person needs to be able to intimately connect as well. In my case, both men have a hard time themselves with 'intimacy'; my husband is very astute at disguising it [the difficulty]."

For Julia, both men in her life had the same world-revolves-around-me orientation as her father did. Each abandoned responsibility. She suffered from all three men because of this. The family unit was threatened in each case [jeopardizing her reigning need crucially, the Moon in Cancer]. Julia had to rescue herself.

Chart 5: "William"

Our final chart in this section (p. 30), belongs to "William."

The analytical outline:

- Some unfinished business (Northern Hemisphere), defensive as well (Eastern Hemisphere).
- Sun-Moon blend: the message needs to be "I am a very deep person, reliable, and right as right; and you must recognize that and know how good I am for you." Excesses of emotional expression show up as the temperamental trappings for well-organized personal opinion and bias. Understanding the motivation behind the thrust for power is very important to success.
- The horoscope seems dominated by Saturn in the 11th—an enormous need for love—and its square to Mercury in Virgo, the final dispositor of the horoscope, *ruler of the 11th.* The emotional excesses promised by the dramatic Sun-Moon blend are going to flow into all kinds of efforts to attract love and allegiance, to have proved to himself that he is lovable, deeply loved.
- Venus in Cancer promises love-relationship needs in a swoon, with love needs hard to be fulfilled, they are so idealized (12th House); additionally, $Venus_{10}$ is quintile (creativity) with Uranus and trine with Neptune, suggesting artistic dimension in the career.
- And further: Venus is quindecile the Node, *introducing a major dimension of "mother" into the emotional love-need mix.*
- There will be a critical time in the family at age thirteen (SA Uranus=MC).

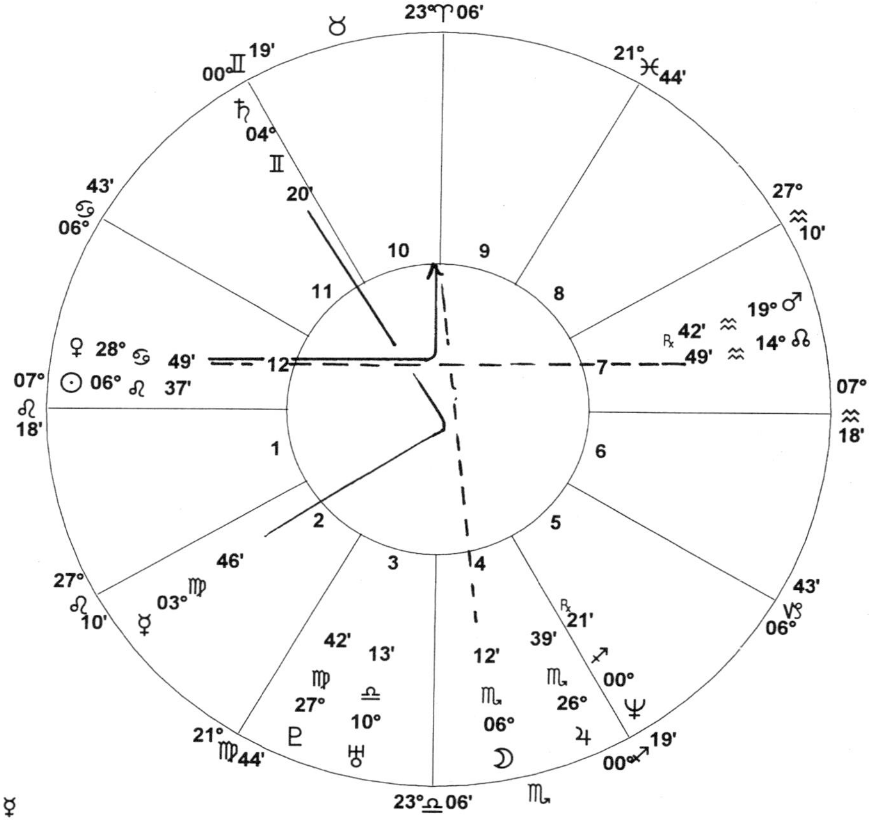

	☽	☉	☿	♀	♂	♃	♄	♅	♆	♇	☊	Mc
☉	□a # 00°25											
☿	✱s 02°26											
♀												
♂		q s 01°54	q a 00°56	#								
♃	II	#		Δs 02°11								
♄	⊼s # 01°52	✱s II 02°17	□a 00°34			#						
♅		✱a 03°37		Qs 00°36		∠a 01°25	Δa 05°54					
♆	II	#	□s 03°25	Δa 01°32		☌a II 03°42	☍s # 03°59					
♇				✱s 01°07		✱s 01°03			✱a 02°39			
☊				q a 01°00	☌a 04°53			Δa 04°35	Qa 02°28	bQa 02°07		
Mc	q s 01°54		II	□a 05°44	✱s 03°24							
Asc	□s # 01°06	☌s II 00°41				#	✱s II 02°58	✱a 02°55	#			

Chart 5

"William"

- William will probably work at home as a freelancer (Moon in the 4th); Moon quindecile Midheaven.

William's father was a passive figure in the early home and his mother was enormously influential. When I asked William if he thought that his mother had favored him, had perhaps transferred affection away from her husband onto him, he replied succinctly, "I was very special to my mother."

When I mentioned about love in a swoon, you could hear his deepest of sighs on the telephone.

With the Sun and Moon square at William's birth, we can expect that his parents *were* in upheaval when he was born; this was so, and the parents split twice over the years, the key time being when William was thirteen.

The Venus appears to share dominance with Saturn: the former serves the latter, with the maternal influence and affection-rewards in early development setting the standards of identity acceptance, the powerful appreciation need established by the Leo Sun and Ascendant.

William feels that he is the antithesis of the person fearing intimacy. To the contrary, he tends to jump immediately—and often too far, in his judgment, too quickly—into deep emotional involvement. "I need that kind of intimacy and depth in a relationship to the point where I seem constitutionally incapable of having a 'light' romance or a casual relationship. I have discovered that I am always seeking my soul-mate and have a strong tendency to settle for nothing less."

William says that this giant need for love has led him often into "wrong relationships," which he did not recognize as such "until it was too late" to extricate himself easily. I suggested to William that his father had not done his job and that the mother had overdone hers, that the balance was out of whack. I also pointed out that perhaps William (at twenty-nine) was meeting women not as mature as he in relationship dynamics.

"Dealing with this aspect of my nature has been a major focus in my life in the last few years."

The difficulty profile in these cases is so common as to become cliché—as mentioned previously, the astrologer must ascertain *to what degree the developmental concerns intrude on the client's self-appreciation and poise in relationship.* Astrologer Erin Sullivan says it well, "The fascinating aspect of the family as an entity [is that] it both enhances and annihilates the individual" growing within it, through it, because of it.[7]

In his *Care of the Soul*, psychotherapist Thomas Moore observes that "In a family you live close to people that otherwise you might not even want to talk to."[8] He goes on to observe as well that the history of the family provides the many images with which a person "is saturated all through adult life." Moore reaches a key point in his discussion, as we have reached here in ours: "What if we thought of the family less as the determining influence by which we are formed and more the raw material from which we can make a life?"

To appreciate this point is to see the beginning of therapy. We must see the family canvas upon which our identity is composed. In the seeing, we must achieve *objectification*. We must learn what we have carried with us from our past development. Then, we must see how fine we are within it all, and **what adjustments we can make in our view of things (mindset) and behavioral patterns in order to present ourselves to the external environment more fulfillingly.**

If we can turn our gaze from looking back, away from blame, we can look forward. We can build anew, or build further upon behaviors that had shown themselves to be effective in the past. We learn to see ourselves in a refreshed image. We stop making the same patterned mistakes, *and we learn to trust who we are.*

When we meet someone, we must know that that "other person" is going through similar developmental tensions. How much does the other person in the relationship trust who he or she is? Can the two of you relate with enough inner self-respect and confidence to show vulnerability, discuss fears,

---

7 Sullivan, *Dynasty*, 28.

8 Moore, *Care of the Soul,* 25.

expose dreams? This ability will define intimacy. And while it is achieved through open, trusting communication, i*t is based upon individual appreciation of Self.*

Henry (p. 23) is learning about himself strongly still. He sees that he is approaching his enormous relationship needs *from his father's perspective* [we might say, *almost inviting* similar letdown and disappointment]. With his understanding, Henry must see himself more as a successful creative businessman (his image for development into the external environment) than as a star-smitten lover (the image from his past development). In this way, as he gains stature through his work, his own company, etc., he gains a refreshed, adult, more mature appreciation of himself and can relate to others more securely. And, most interestingly, Henry will begin to attract more relationships with other, more mature people.

For Frances (p. 15), her keen intelligence (Mercury in Gemini conjunct Venus in Gemini, ruling the 3rd) will help her free herself from past patterning. Becoming an astrologer, with skills particularly enriched by her having lived through so much of this difficult patterning, will give her an ever-broadening humanitarian base upon which to see how fine a person she is. Her problem will then become setting an example for her husband who is mired in similar aloneness and developmental difficulty.

Ruth (p. 19), has already made the transition. It took her and her patient, loving mate three years to accomplish intimacy. It worked, and she can now allow intimacy to energize her relationship and life even further.

Julia (p. 26), our last case, turned her attention to her husband. There is hope. Her quest was not simply to throw it all to the wind and to avoid repeating her mistake yet once again in another marriage, but *to appreciate how she has survived that process to date*, how secure she had now become within herself, and how she could use that as a way to be helpful to her husband and others. Unfortunately this effort failed, and we will study Julia's divorce astrology in chapter 6.

Intimacy *is* the revelation of the most inner Self, without fear. It can only be accomplished through "being a friend to yourself," as Thomas Moore so nicely puts it.[9] When that inner friendship is not there, when the developmental weights and short circuits have not been recognized, inspected, and adjusted, we often cannot tolerate the self-criticism we have been patterned to feel, and we project it onto our relationships [recall Ruth's projection (chart 2) of her father-upset onto her mate]. *The difficulties in relationships so often mask, so often echo relationships with ourselves.*

French essayist Michel Montaigne said it most penetratingly, some 400 years ago: "The distance between us and others is the same as the distance between us and ourselves."

---

9 Moore, *Soul Mates,* 24.

2
INTIMACY
Needs in Relationships

All our behaviors are organized to help us fulfill our needs. There are the subsidiary needs *to think* a particularly individual way, *to relate* a certain way, *to apply* our energy a certain way, etc. All of these subsidiary needs (faculties of behavior) work together as best they can to fulfill the grand *reigning need* of the personality, symbolized by the Moon. Each individual has this palette of colors with which to portray her or his personality. When two people begin to relate to each other, *two need profiles meet.*

To discuss this complicated meeting, let's first explore an individual's need profile in more detail. Let me use my horoscope (chart 6), since I know it best.

Chart 6: Noel Tyl

Capricorn (administratively organized and driving) energy fuels my reigning need to be dramatic, expressive, and appreciated for it by everyone with whom I am in contact (the Moon in Leo, ruling the Ascendant; the Sun in the 7th conjoined with Jupiter, p. 36). All my behavioral faculties will, at one time or another, more frequently than not, be conscripted to fulfill that reigning need.

My need to think a certain way is keyed by Mercury in Capricorn—I like to say that *I need to hear the grass grow!* In other words, my mind

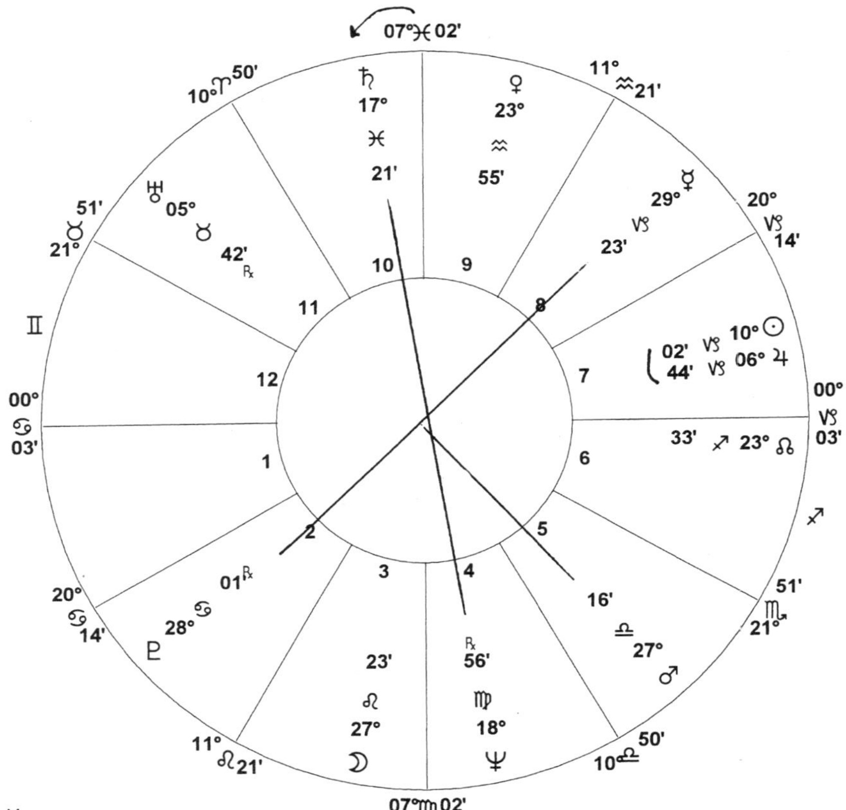

	☽	☉	☿	♀	♂	♃	♄	♅	♆	♇	☊	Mc
☉	⚼s 02°21											
☿	⚻a 02°00											
♀	☍s 03°28	∠a 01°07										
♂	✶s 00°07	Qs 00°46	□s 02°07	△a 03°21								
♃		☌s ∥ 03°19		∠s 02°11								
♄						Qs 01°23						
♅		△s 04°21		Qs 00°13		△s 01°02						
♆							☍a 01°36	⚼a 01°45				
♇		#	☍s 01°23		□a 00°44	#						
☊	△s 03°50	∥		✶s 00°22	✶s 03°44	∥			□a 04°37	#		
Mc	#	✶a 03°01			∥	✶s 00°18		✶s 01°20			Qs 01°29	
Asc	✶s 02°40	#	⚻s 00°39		△s 02°46	☍a # 06°41				∥	☍s # 06°30	

Chart 6

Noel Tyl

Dec. 31, 1936, 03:57 P.M. EST, West Chester, Pennsylvania

75W36, 39N57

likes to work with incisive, detailed understanding. If I am put in a position where that kind of thinking can not prevail, then I am a fish out of water.

Of course, a complementary view of the mindset and individual communication style for anyone comes from the 3rd House, which is pretty dramatic here in my case. The Moon in the 3rd almost always suggests the middle-person, the go-between, the persuasive, selling nature. Here, holding my Leo Moon, ruler of the Ascendant (with the ruler of the 3rd, the Sun, conjoined with Jupiter), the communication is decidedly dramatic, emotional, and probably aimed at making a personal imprint on things. If I cannot do that, I am frustrated.

The Venus-in-Aquarius position suggests a humanitarian way of relating, and it certainly falls into the individual portrait being assembled: the public communicator, the powerful emotional thrust (00 Cancer, "Aries Point" Ascendant), the Moon in the 3rd in Leo with the Venus in opposition (full awareness). The Venus adds *acceptability* to the other strong, possibly overbearing features.

Indeed, there are so many more manifestations within this network of symbols—my career in opera, my international life-experience, etc.—but, staying with our intimacy discussion, we must now assess the inhibition potential within relationships that is symbolized by my Saturn, ruler of the 7th, opposed by Neptune, and how this can be tied to my public image.

Indeed, there is the break-up in my early home (SA MC=Saturn; Neptune rules the 10th and opposes natal Saturn; the opposition is within the parental axis; Mercury, ruler of the parental 4th, is opposed by Pluto and squared by Mars). Indeed, with the great need to be appreciated and honored, the sense of my need to be dominant in a relationship (to lead it) is clear. Therefore, for relationships to offer the opportunity for intimacy, my self-identifying need press must not be jeopardized, *it must not be questioned*. Certainly there can be feelings shared by two self-respecting parties that will lead to behavioral adjustments for intercompatibility, but disrespect for anyone's need network is intolerable. The point of intimacy is that divergent views or feelings or behaviors *can* be discussed—and that is a goal of intimate relationships—**without any fear of the core being assailed, of one being "put down," of being criticized, rejected, or abandoned.**

Now, there are other considerations as well: the expansive, may I say benevolent, Sun-Jupiter conjunction in the 7th may offset much of the Saturn rulership of the 7th. Does this suggest that I the professional, the performer, if you will, will make this grand impact with the public but remain somehow alone privately? Are those the two sides of the coin? That would be a very keen and worthwhile insight. This is a nice way of saying there is a one-on-one relationship difficulty that must be faced on the road to maturation.

The questions begged then would be "Just how much 'performance' is necessary to prove Self, to fulfill the imposing need for appreciation and honor? Why is it so extreme?" In a consultation with you, I might begin by saying, "Yes, it is that strong, and I remember when my parents did not come to see the big championship basketball game in which I starred . . . and it was only fifteen minutes from where we lived!" This reply carries enormous emotional content with it—even now, forty-five years later. Appreciating my need profile, one sees that my reply was certainly not a non sequitur.

I could then add, "And they never came to see me perform in an opera!"[10]

The Mars position in Libra—in addition to the Venus in Aquarius—probably helps me to be acceptable to the world rather than in a fight with it. *The energy here loves peace.* I see five sides to very issue; a very good trait in a peaceful, self-confident relationship effort. In maturity now, I have eased off controlling details and driving my career full-steam ahead. Yes, I have achieved much, but at the same time, perspectives have adjusted themselves around just what *is* important.

Mars squares the axis of Pluto-Mercury. This is intense communication power in a no-axe-to-grind way. Note that the powerful Moon is sextile with

---

10 While my sainted (step)father supported me superbly in every way, his allegiance to my mother was demanded by her complicated, years-long neuroses. She is the Neptune in my 4th. He never could get away from that.

the Mars. All of that T-square of perception is funneled supportively into the communication power network through the Moon in the 3rd.

Already, within these few paragraphs outlining the barest elements of the horoscope, *we understand what will be required within relationship.* We understand what this man brings into a relationship, what his needs are, what his vulnerabilities are.

Now, I could pick someone with whom I am in relationship, analyze similarly that person's basic need profile, and relate that profile to mine. This is true-life *synastry*: the relation of one individual, one horoscope, to another. **The only practicable way to accomplish synastry—chart comparison—is in terms of needs, *not in terms of averaged mathematics.*** [11]

For example: my creative thrust is definitely keyed by the Mars complex, the way it brings the mind, perception, etc. into the communication arena of the 3rd House. If I am with someone in a relationship (work or personal) whose Saturn, for example, is positioned at 25–29 Aries, my being will feel it. I will feel controlled, disapproved of. Immediately, one sees the potential intrusion upon my self-image within the relationship. Sure, I believe I'm mature enough to weather the storm, but for how long? To what depth?

"Weathering the storm" is a Mars-in-Libra statement; even a Venus-in-Aquarius statement. And we can see in my horoscope that Mars and Venus are in an easy trine. This certainly brings grace to the whole issue, doesn't it?

So, when we bring ourselves to the relationship moment, as we work to know our Self well, *to gain the secure composure of safety with showing our strengths **and** vulnerabilities to someone else,* **we must know as well the need profile of the person to whom we are relating.**

11 It is the dehumanization by numbers and measurement systems that underlines the failure of composite and averaging charting. When computer resourcefulness came to astrology, computational power was brought into every possible consideration in astrological measurement. Bringing two charts/individuals together in that way did/does not work.

The Inner Planets

The inner planets Mercury, Venus, and Mars are the most responsive of our planet symbols. They receive stimulus; they suggest how our minds, emotions, and energies will then react to situations and to pressure. Together they suggest how our inner environment relates to the outer environment. They lead the way to fulfillment of the reigning need of the personality, symbolized by the Moon in *its* sign.

♂ In the external environment, Mars in the Fire signs suggests pioneering, deploying aggression in Aries; getting away with murder in Leo; or exploiting arch-opinionation in Sagittarius. When aspects do not *modify* these positions, they can represent energies that are very hard to bear in relationships. These energies are strongly ego-orientated. Our society's gender profiles make these positions very difficult for women to express easily: the aggressive woman, the winning woman, the opinionated woman is *not yet* at a premium in our culture, even though, within the sense of equal opportunity in the marketplace, times may be changing ever so slowly.

Mars in the Water Signs for a man or woman suggests running the home, exploiting emotional power in Cancer; using passion, criticism, or sexuality as a control strategy in Scorpio; or censoring, holding back, being cautious, even diluting energy in Pisces. These positions can appear more supportive, energizing, or ameliorating in relationships. But we must remember that if these symbols are strongly modified, we can gain the dysfunction of too much emotional power, too much controlling energy, too much weakness or passivity.

Mars in the Air Signs suggests in Libra being judiciously even-handed, but prepared to upset the apple cart when push comes to shove; making things happen creatively and individualistically for others in Aquarius; or extreme diversification in Gemini. These positions seem to fare the best in our culture within the altruism demanded of relationships.

Mars in the Earth signs suggests making things happen emphatically, in one's own way, in Capricorn; sticking tenaciously to what has been built up in Taurus; or mastering the technique of whatever is important in Virgo. These positions embody a very high level of competition and effectiveness.

Showing one's energy to others in definitive style is very important; it should be showing one at one's best. Any frustration to this energy can drive a hot poker into the core of being. The husband who does not listen to his wife's opinions if she has Mars in Sagittarius is causing enormous frustration for his wife and undermining their relationship together; and vice versa, of course.

How does the Leo (or Mars in Leo) wife relate to the Leo (or Mars in Leo) husband—or vice versa? How did they get together in the first place? I remember vividly a Leo couple coming to me at a party and asking something like, "Tell us about us!" He was a prominent bank officer in one of the biggest banks in the world, and socially it seemed that she did all the talking; he was a picture of restrained monumentality. I simply asked in return, "Who leads?" And *that* was a moment. My remark brought forward the confrontation of their individual need systems. The wife was not as unnerved as her husband, who seethed silently as I thought of a way to relax the tension for them.

My Mars dimension might be very well *appreciated* [there's my word again!] in relationship since it is nonthreatening. But should I meet with a Mars in Aries or Mars in Sagittarius or in Leo, I am hard-pressed to endure being second-fiddle to that more powerful energy thrust; the Moon in Leo, fueled by the Capricorn Sun, can not take that easily, without much accommodation. There cannot easily be an intimate relationship on that wavelength *unless* I am internally sure of my identity (my Moon in Leo) and *also sure that my vulnerability (Mars in Libra) will not be attacked or exploited by someone.* With that composure—*knowing I am established enough*—I can then selflessly and openly applaud and embrace the identity of someone else.

When Mars is peregrine, it will usually dominate the horoscope and must be given a wide berth, so to speak, as it searches for attachment, connection, inclusion, a role in life development. When it is retrograde, the energy will seem to go in before it will go out; the question is why? For censorship, editing, checking, caution, habit . . . usually shying away from early reprisals?

Going Further

When we see Mars in Scorpio, Sagittarius, or Capricorn we must know that these positions are suggesting very difficult energy positions within society's mandate to relate peacefully and fairly. It is extremely difficult for people with such energies to fit into relationships easily, without careful, conscious amelioration. This is especially so for a woman in our society, since Martian energies (along with the Sun) are so-called masculine energies.

Mars in Scorpio: explosive emotional coercion, relentless determination, often with strategic sexual overtones as well (Bobby Kennedy, Mao Tse-Tung, Eleanor Roosevelt, Joseph Goebels, Sammy Davis, Jr.).

Mars in Sagittarius: arch-opinionation, demanding independence, unable to stop and smell the roses (Oscar Wilde, Richard Nixon, Billy Graham, Judy Garland).

Mars in Capricorn: working for ambitious fulfillment; the use of weaponry; threat and reprisal possible (Thomas Edison, Dwight Eisenhower, Ronald Reagan, Theodore Roosevelt).

We can appreciate that these Mars positions will relate most easily with the Sun or Moon in Water, Fire, or Earth, respectively. That trine relationship will usually then add fuel flow to the Mars turbine. It is formidable.

I feel that Mars leads the way for us for the most part: we have to initiate activity to get a process started that will fulfill our needs. How we do that—at what expense, often—will be suggested by the Mars position. Yassir Arafat has his Mars in Libra (!), which is apparently antithetical to his image of a driving revolutionary. His Mars is peregrine, dominating his being; the search for Libran parity obsesses him. And let us remember it is he who extended his hand at the signing of the Israel-PLO peace accord. Beyond peace, we must say that Arafat is for *fairness*, from his point of view, a prime focus of "work-for-the-underdog" Libra. Arafat can not be ordering the hidden violence that infests the land/peace negotiations; he may be forced to overlook it, but he is not planning or ordering it.

Bill Clinton has his Mars in Libra as well; it is the central focus of his charisma and more. The Mars is camouflaged and softened by the exact conjunction with Neptune; Venus is nearby; Venus is the final dispositor in Libra and establishes a feminine-sensitive profile, in concert with the Moon in Taurus.[12]

♀ With Venus, we have the symbol for how we need to relate to be most efficient. Venus-in-Aries was named "the Amazon flirt" by Evangeline Adams; the flirtatiousness (man or woman) is to test the waters, to see if one is attractive, desirable; it is *not* so just to make constant conquests. Venus in Leo is self-dramatizing, even to the point of emotional theatricality (should aspects push it this way); there can be a kind of pageantry brought to the aesthetics of relationship. In Sagittarius, Venus very often arches above everything: the presence of the emotional needs and how these needs are to be satisfied are often imposing concerns with which to deal, sometimes cerebrated to the philosophical.

Venus in Cancer needs to be in a lush blanketing of comfort, in a swoon (see William, chart 5, p. 30); in Scorpio, deeply involved with primal values; and in Pisces, part of a poetical ideal that blends in anywhere.

Venus in Libra needs to be lovelier than lovely in interrelationships; in Aquarius, humane and extended to many, caring for the world; or in Gemini, cerebrated, thought about more than acted upon.

Venus in Capricorn, as we have seen, suggests that more time than normal is needed for emotional development [find out why!]; in Taurus, that there is the need for faithfulness—for good or bad—for it to prevail as a badge of identity; or in Virgo where Venus can suggest keen efficiency in managing things emotional, talking about emotions without (or before) feeling them.

---

12 Bill Clinton: August 9, 1946 at 8:51 A.M. CST in Hope, Arkansas.

When Venus is peregrine, the life turns on a *relational* pivot (and the Houses it rules dominate experience). When it is retrograde, emotional fulfillment is not easily forthcoming; there is something else involved, a second agenda, that is getting in the way, usually seen through other aspect structures. [In a woman's horoscope, Venus retrograde is most often more difficult to deal with than it is in a man's horoscope, because of the higher premium paid to emotional expression for a woman within the societal stereotypes.] Venus retrograde becomes very important within sexuality concerns in relationships, as we shall see. It is a very difficult developmental consideration.

Venus, along with the Moon, defines the feminine in our society.

Going Further

We know that Venus is never more than 44 degrees from the Sun. The probability of its being in the same sign as the Sun is high. This tells us that our Sun, much more often than not, is symbolically influencing our needs to relate, our way of relating with core-characteristic invigoration. When Venus is *not* in the same sign as the Sun, we are dealing with something more interesting, if you will; another dimension. Venus in Aquarius relates differently than Venus in Capricorn, clearly. The Aquarius position for the Capricorn's Venus will try to brighten things conspicuously. The Aries Sun's Venus in Pisces will tend to tone things down in personal presentation for relationship. Here we would find a special grace or a poignant vulnerability.

Since Mercury is never farther from the Sun than 23 degrees, Mercury is more often than not in the same sign as the Sun. When our need to think a certain way is imbued with our Sun energy *and* with our style of relating, i.e., when the Sun, Mercury, and Venus are in conjunction, an idealism is focused and pronounced. Our innermost faculties are tightly illuminated, even burnt up (*combusta*), as anorexia is a healthy body figure idealized to extreme and run amuck; we can expect any kind of fanaticism. **Idealism points up where we are most vulnerable, the area in our life wherein grief is most often felt.** With our growing understanding of intimacy, it is clear that, with the triple conjunction of Sun, Mercury, and Venus, **intimacy must begin with the security and sharing of *this point of idealization.***

The idealization formation occurs as well with Sun conjunct Venus, with Sun conjunct Mercury, with Mercury conjunct Venus (or in mutual reception), only the intensity (the grip) is apparently less. When the Mercury-Venus conjunction occurs in the sign not holding the Sun, we have an idealizing dimension focused within an entirely different energy field than that symbolized by the Sun. In any case, the analyst's question must be how the idealization structures defend the personality; against what is the defense necessary; how much energy is being used up in defense; is defense so necessary now in adulthood?

When Sun, Venus, and Mercury find themselves in *three different signs*, the fragmentation of the inner identity formation is obvious. It is difficult for the person to "get it together," to make the identity presentation that is organized for intimacy in relationship. Jerry Lewis, the great comedian, director, writer, philanthropist (March 16, 1926 at 12:15 P.M. in Newark, New Jersey; see chart 8, p. 58), has the Sun in Pisces (conjoined with Uranus, his extraordinary, intense emotional sensitivity), Mercury in Aries square Pluto (the mind afire with perception), and Venus in Aquarius conjunct Jupiter (the benevolent humanitarian). Mercury and Venus are in sextile—a rare aspect—which brings out the idealism we have just been discussing in relation to Mercury-Venus-(Sun) contacts. This gifted man's diversification is extraordinary, and the personal identity fragmentation within it certainly a cross for him to bear.

☿ Mercury symbolizes how our minds need to work, how we communicate to be maximally efficient. In Fire signs, the mental energy needs to be heated, argumentative, showy; in the Water signs, it needs very strong orientation to the emotional well-being; in Air, it leans to what others think, how they will react to what one offers; in Earth, development is usually absorbed with tactics to make progress.

Mercury peregrine will dominate the horoscope (see how Julia's mind, p. 26, did such a good job of stabilizing her relationship problems. It's fair to say she substituted thinking for feeling within her family dilemma. The objective will be to guide her husband's growth into such security). Mercury retrograde suggests a second agenda, some other line of developmental concern, most often related to the reigning need of the horoscope (the Moon) and to frustration in early homelife development.

We will add more to the study of the inner planets in chapter 3, in relation to *animus* and *anima* dimensions of identity and the fears we face in relationship

Two Need Profiles Together: Synastry

As soon as two individuals begin to relate, a bonding starts that is involved with reciprocal resource exchange: *what can you do for me and what can I do for you.*

Social psychologists call this a *gain-loss* process. In our discussion, we are seeing one person's need profile relating to another person's need profile: each is trying to help the other fulfill personally orientated needs because of the reward that may be/are at the end of the process.

For this process of resource exchange to work well, there must be **a frustration tolerance in each person for those needs that are *not* well satisfied in the relationship (loss), and an appreciation for the reward gain from those needs that *are* well satisfied (gain).** Then, individual self-respect and confidence—with no fear of reprisal from the other person—allow intimacy to begin with the other individual in the relationship.

In the simplest of terms, the need fulfillment process within relationship and the possible introduction of intimacy come down to the bare but enormously challenging truth: **I can only be intimate with someone when I can be myself without fear.**

We must not forget our discussion to this point: the astrological delineation (appreciation) of individual needs is unavoidably filtered through the development experience in the early homelife. There are always mitigating circumstances; there are always different degrees of need development. There are always different levels of fulfillment and frustration, each spawning other behaviors within the identifying pattern.

A young male client with whom I consulted this morning has the Sun in Aquarius and the Moon in Aries: a reigning need tremendously orientated to ego prominence (to be *numero uno*), to place himself into prominence through self-awareness, keen thought, and a judicial attitude about the rest of the world. We can see his Sun-Moon positions as those of a natural and genuine superiority complex.

The young man's Mars was in Capricorn, Venus was in Pisces, and Mercury was in Aquarius—*feel* those positions in terms of behavioral needs—all of which start to channel his development into getting something done for others . . . *in order to gain ego importance.*

But there were mitigating circumstances indeed: his mother was a prostitute (corroborated by $Neptune_4$ conjunct the Node) who gave him up after a few years to a distant, resentful father ($Saturn_{Rx}$). My client discovered himself by learning to fight obstreperously at school, by turning to thievery, by finally dropping out of school. He never understood the boundaries of behavior (a Moon-in-Aries extremism) until some large Plutonic transits paralleled alteration of his perspectives away from rebellion and put him on track to real-life achievement and development. He is now a model young businessman, and his having learned the hard way—having triumphed in spite of all the impediments—has given him a poise and confidence that are extraordinary.

In our society, we hear often about relationships, "Well, I'm the live wire and he's the strong silent type," or, "She understands my need to be the life of the party." We hear as well, "Opposites attract," with the implication being that, "Similars are boring or off-putting."

Psychological studies show that this is a complicated issue. Some investigators find that married couples tend to have *complementary* need systems and others find that married couples tend to have *similar* need systems.

Esteemed psychology professor Elliot Aronson thinks that it all depends on which personality characteristics are under consideration.[13]

The "Odd Couple," bringing together someone obsessively neat and someone gladly sloppy, probably will not work out. It is strongly suggested that two neat people will relate—or twsimilars attracting each other. But consider this: the extrovert may need the introvert as an audience, but how easily will nights-on-the-town be repeatedly sacrificed to a stay-at-home preference? Within need systems, there is a ranking of degrees. It is complicated.

What if a male is highly nurturing—a Cancerian dimension predominating, for example—and is partnered with a woman who is archly independent? This relationship might bring misery, *unless* there were something else that was highly valued, the fulfillment of which was *more important* than the nurturing dimension. Very often in difficult need-profile interaction, the sexuality dimension can upset the balance decidedly. This may be the offsetting—but rarely long-lasting—reward.

Additionally, there is the family filter through which the extravert has passed (behaviors that have been routined to gain parental attention?) and the introvert as well (behaviors suppressed through repeated criticism?). The two have found a way to turn off the overcompensation and share long-needed respect and support. Maybe that is how the relationship will work.

And finally, we must remember the forces of societal expectation and approval: in our culture, men are supposed to be relatively dominant and wives to be relatively submissive in relationships. Aronson reports that *when the needs of a couple work out to coincide with the role norms set forth by society*, the chances of marital happiness are increased. This suggests that the male is being himself and the female is being herself, and *the predictable, reliable approval of others around them reinforces this behavior.* The couple's behaviors and opinions are molded by the explicit and implicit approval of others, by society in general.

---

13 Aronson, 388–397.

Another question: how can relationships that begin apparently so well start to fall apart? The evaluation, "My wife doesn't understand me!" certainly was *not* the case heading into the wedding! "He's just so stupid; everything he does [overstatement, of course] is wrong," certainly was not the case during the initial attraction and the early years of marriage when the couple did so many wonderful things together and the husband was so successful. *What has changed?*

We know that Uranian contact with the Ascendant (by Arc or by Transit) tends to suggest disruption in relationship (the Ascendant is one end of the personal horizon, remember; the other end is relationships).[14] In more complete terms, **the Uranian influence accentuates the individual at the expense of the relationship.** Perhaps that *is* what is behind the sense of "Well, we just outgrew each other" or "We are now heading into separate directions." The individual ascends above or past the relationship in the focus of gain and loss, of need pressure and fulfillment. A greater effort is made *for the Self,* and that effort is rewarded *away from the relationship*.

Psychologists note a "dark side" to long-term relationships that can also help us to understand change. The solidarity at the beginning of a relationship is undoubtedly graced by intimacy: "The priceless comfort of being accepted by someone who knows your shortcomings as well as your strengths." Aronson suggests that, once we have grown certain of the rewarding behavior of a person, *that person may become less powerful as a source of reward than a stranger can be.* By the same token, a loved one has great potential as a punisher.[15]

It has been found in psychological testing that there is a tendency for people *to react more positively to strangers than to friends* when either group was

14 Indeed there are other key measurements that suggest this as well [Outer Planet fourth harmonic Arc or Transit relationship with the Sun/Moon midpoint; high tension by Arc or Transit with the ruler of the 7th, etc.], but the Uranus example supports the idea of our discussion here best.

15 We can note the lyrics of so many popular songs; e.g., "Some Enchanted Evening," for the rewarding stranger; "You Always Hurt the One You Love," for the punisher.

designated as the source of relatively positive evaluation of the subjects.[16] The perhaps over-familiar compliment from the spouse carries much more impact *when presented by a stranger*, and, in turn, one's liking for the stranger is increased.

Aronson's comment is that we seem to be forever seeking favor in the eyes of strangers while, at the same time, we are being hurt by friends and other familiar people. This tells us that our appreciation of the stranger is a kind of *speeded up intimacy process*, with the key being that the stranger, the friends "out there," **do not know our vulnerabilities**. We are meeting strangers quickly, looking and being our best, and there is this marvelous compliment that lifts us high! We rarely doubt or discredit it.[17] This certainly is a rationale for the allure of prostitution as well.

This appreciation for the stranger through the positive statement or act is a vital energy that also occurs *within the astrological consultation*. I have long noticed that when I paid a compliment to a client, I have sometimes received enormous appreciation for it. I have then asked, "Hasn't your wife/husband told you this recently?" [I add the word "recently" as a grace, implying that "of course she/he knows this positive observation and has told you many times before."] Through this kind of subtle bonding within the ego-appreciation process of the astrological consultation, much client strengthening can be accomplished.

Gains in esteem are essential to a relationship that is continuing to grow. Fresh ways of communicating this are exciting ways to reassure the process toward intimacy.

And lastly, we must know that we tend to relate better with people *when bonded through disclosure,* when they *honor* us by revealing something intimate *and negative* about themselves. This is especially true when the person is

---

16 O. J. Harvey (1962), "Personality factors in resolution of conceptual incongruities." *Sociometry,* 25, 336-352.

17 Unless we have severe self-worth anxieties and have taught ourselves that nothing good about us is acceptable or believable.

normally reserved. The implication is that there is something special about *us* that made him or her feel like opening up. This is the "best friend" with whom one *can* be intimate, while intimacy may be difficult with the spouse.[18] And here again, during the astrological consultation, we encounter similar dynamics connected with disclosure.[19]

Interplanetary Relationships

Running through these large concepts is the actual planetary interrelationships from one person to another, from one horoscope to another. We appreciate as best we can the need structure and early development patterning in one horoscope, appreciate the same in another, and then seek out the specific contacts between them to punctuate the commonsense assessment we are making about relationship potential.

For example: Man A has the Sun in Virgo and the Moon in Taurus. The Sun's position is modified by a strong conjunction with Neptune. The Sun-Moon blend suggests an emotional tie-in with materialism, with acquisition to define identity. The Neptune dimension adds vision and/or illusory dimensions; i.e., is it real, is it reliable?

Man B has the Sun in Aquarius and the Moon in Capricorn. The Sun's position is modified by very powerful squares from Mars, Saturn, and Uranus in Taurus. The Sun-Moon blend suggests people-orientated energy focused administratively through the sense of bureaucratic expediency. These are the positions of a public leader, the rugged individualistic campaigner who sways the crowd and makes things happen. This is a tough, hard-driving image.

When we note that Man A has his Taurus Moon right in the middle of everything in Man B's tension network, his Saturn and Uranus conjunct Man A's Moon, you can feel the tension extremely clearly.

---

18 Skotko, P. K. (1981). "The relation between interpersonal attraction and measures of self-disclosure." *Journal of Social Psychology,* 112, 311–312. Et al.

19 Please see Tyl, *The Creative Astrologer*, beginning with page 87.

Man A is Yassir Arafat (August 27, 1929) and Man B is Ehud Barak (February 12, 1942), prime minister of Israel during the outbreak of civil war in Israel 1999–2001. Additionally, Arafat's Moon, as the focal horoscope for the Palestinian Liberation Front, is exactly conjunct the national Sun of Israel (suggesting two halves of a once-unified land).

There is primal tension here. It is undeniable. It is probably insoluble.[20] One of these men will have to absent the negotiations for any progress to be made.

When Mars, Uranus, or Pluto in one horoscope relates to the Sun, Moon, Mercury, Venus, or Mars of a second horoscope, the synastric process relating the need profile of two individuals becomes extremely important. There will be an attack, an enflaming, or a power-competitive aggravation placed on a need-focus in the other person. The relationship easily bristles at the affront.

But we must keep in mind that, if the Mars is weakened somehow in the one person, it will be *less* aggravating, clearly. Pope John Paul II has Mars in Libra, retrograde (!), and Peregrine (!!); his Mars will not be aggravating if it squares, conjoins, or opposes the other person's Sun, Moon, Mercury, Venus, or Mars. It *could be* just the opposite, with the other person's Mars (or Uranus or Pluto) aggravating Pope John Paul's system! And the point is made: the weakened Mars exposes a *vulnerability*. In the quest for intimacy, acknowledgement and management of this vulnerability with secure poise is vitally important.

When Saturn in one person's horoscope relates to the inner planets of another person's horoscope, there is the sense of control, delay, or depression [Arafat's relationship with Barak, above].

When the aspecting planet is Neptune, there is the potential of sharing imagination, deluding, deceiving, or inspiring; there is no way to be sure; reality will tell.

---

20 Astrology could be so helpful in planning strategies and productive interpersonal relations in government diplomacy.

When Pluto is involved, there is usually a very strong competition for power in terms of the planet receiving the Plutonic onslaught—or there is empowerment offered in assistance. If the person receiving the Pluto aspect recognizes the need for support and empowerment in terms of his/her Sun, Moon, Mercury, Venus, or Mars, the person sending the aspect may be well received indeed.

Needs We Do Not Understand: The Nodes

People in intimate, harmonious, productive relationships often feel that their relationship was "made in heaven," that "they were destined for each other." That's what clients are looking for when they ask astrologers about meeting their *soul mate*. Here in our discussion, we should ask if there is a special dimension within our astrology that can embellish horoscopic need-profiles with this soul mate dimension?

The sense of "soul mate" implies strongly that two people have been together before. This introduces the thought of previous lives. Where else, how else could one soul have "mated" with another, find and recognize another now? Within the reference to soul mates, there is the sense that souls are hunting for each other, to complete something somehow.

I have long observed a fascinating synastric tie: whenever there is a tight relationship, usually conjunction/opposition or square between one person's Lunar Nodal Axis and another person's planet, Ascendant, or Midheaven, there is a dimension to the relationship tie that goes very, very deep. The relationship can even be strange, developing itself into hard-to-understand directions. The relationship can drain someone's resources, even possess someone, tying two people together, come hell or high water! The relationship can be inspiring.

Astrologer Jeffrey Green, innovator of Evolutionary Astrology, approaches the same finding. He writes, "When Pluto or another planet is squaring the Nodal Axis of another person, an evolutionary and karmic condition exists wherein those two people have had prior life connections in which something has occurred that has caused a separation to occur between them. Thus, the relationship has been interrupted—it has not come to completion. The intention in this life is to repeat those conditions or situations in this life in order for the relationship to move forwards—to evolve and resolve."[21]

Fascinating ideas.

I have noted that when the Sun or Moon is involved with another person's Nodal Axis, there seems to be a core recognition, a sense of belonging to one another, if you will. Even under the worst of circumstances, the relationship bond is hard to break. When Mercury is involved, the relationship bond is powerfully focused in the mind, in the thinking process, in communication.

With Venus, romanticism; with Mars, aggression or defensiveness, and strong sexuality; with Jupiter, enthusiasm, understanding, learning; with Saturn, control, manipulation; with Uranus, intense, electrifying magnetism; with Neptune, deception, mistrust, or we see fantasy and aesthetics shared; with Pluto, there is empowerment and climactic resolve. The Midheaven involvement links one person to the other often in terms of career, or a sense of personal destiny; with the Ascendant, the focus is how one is presented to the world, one's image possibly being more important than one's real substance.

Chart 7: Hitler/Braun Double-Ring Horoscope

One of history's most improbable relationships was Adolph Hitler, born April 20, 1889 at around 6:30 P.M., LMT in Braunau, Austria, and Eva Braun, born February 6, 1912 at around 3:25 A.M., CET in Munich, Germany (p. 55). Hitler was chancellor of Germany, der Fuehrer (the Leader); Braun was an uneducated and, some say, a distant cousin of Hitler, twenty-three years his junior. They were tied together from remote levels of the social spectrum, in strange ways, and finally married the day before committing suicide together deep underground in a besieged Berlin bunker (April 29, 1945). Eva Braun's Nodal Axis at 25 Aries-Libra was exactly conjunct Hitler's Mercury at 25 Aries, *which was positioned conjunct his horizon axis, on the cusp of his 7th House!*

---

21 Green, 15.

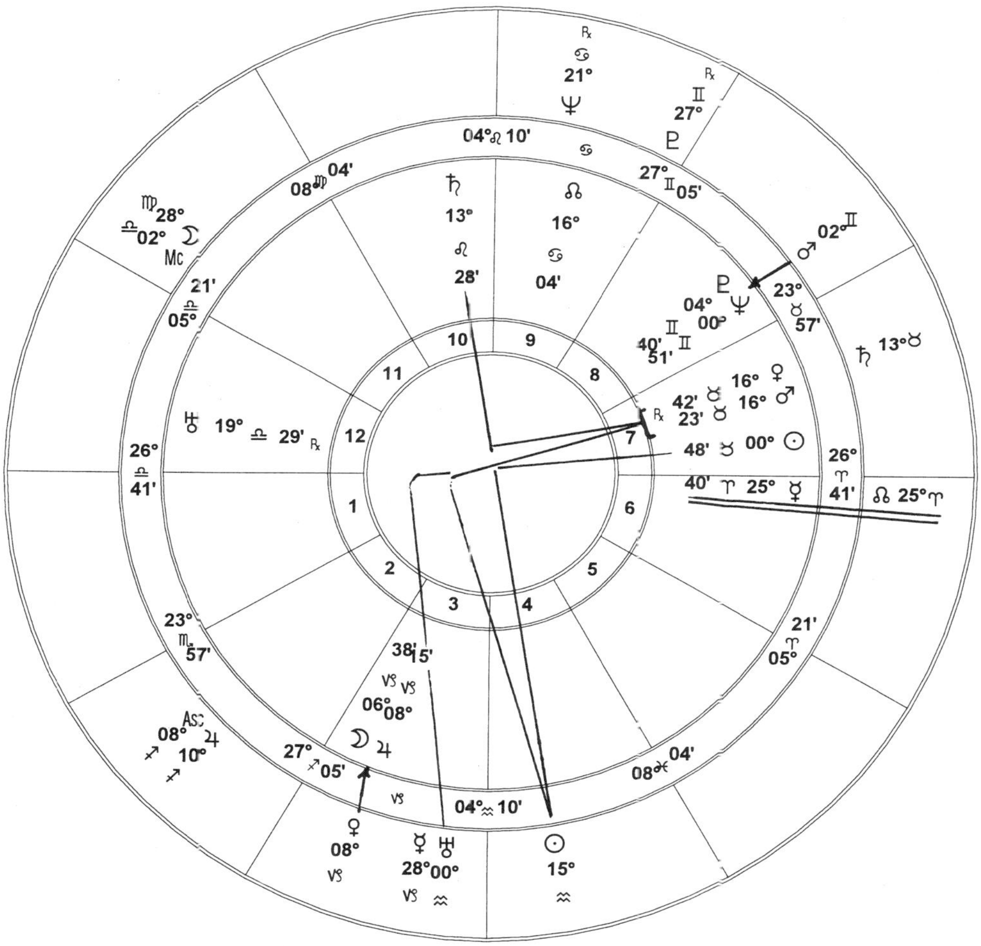

Chart 7

Inner Chart
Adolf Hitler
April 20, 1889, 6:30 A.M. LMT
Braunau am Inn, Austria
13E02, 48N15

Outer Chart
Eva Braun
Feb. 6, 1912, 3:25 A.M. CET
Munich, Germany
13E02, 48N15

There was much more: Braun's Sun in Aquarius was square Hitler's exact Venus-Mars conjunction in Taurus. Many psychohistorical analysts have ascribed deep sexual problems to Hitler, and here we see Braun's involvement with them—Hitler's Saturn, square to his Venus-Mars conjunction, opposed Braun's Sun; her Mars square his Sun/Moon midpoint: they seem tied together in a sadomasochistic drama. Her Uranus was square to Hitler's Sun exactly, "electrifying" him. And even further, we can see Braun's Venus conjunct Hitler's Moon and Jupiter, a tie through beauty and appreciation of it; her Mars conjunct his Pluto, her tie to his empowering presence. This pair came together in ways and purposes we simply can not understand. The bond was overwhelmingly, inexorably confirmed by the nodal contact with Hitler's mind, his Mercury.

I feel it safe to conjecture that *without* the nodal contact between them, these two people would have been more than happy to be far, far away from each other: the other synastric measurements would not have been organized under the cloak of the Nodal contact; they would have been disruptive to efficient living.

A fascinating example of the touch of fate, if you will, is in the coming together of Sirhan Sirhan (March 19, 1944) and Robert Kennedy (November 20, 1925), on Kennedy's day of death, June 6, 1968. The assassin's Nodal Axis was at 5 Leo-Aquarius *exactly square* the candidate's strident and critical Mars in Scorpio! Imagine the imposing, inflaming energy Sirhan felt from Kennedy and his campaign issues; how all that long occupied Sirhan's mind, leading him to assassinate the senator. Was this a conclusion of some tension founded in a previous life?

Richard Rodgers (June 28, 1902), the famed Broadway musical composer, had his Lunar Nodal Axis at 1 Scorpio tightly conjunct lyricist Oscar Hammerstein's Saturn at 0 Scorpio (July 12, 1895). This tells us for sure that, in their collaboration, the words came first, before the music; Rodgers was receiving Hammerstein's eloquent leadership! Additionally, Hammerstein's Nodal Axis at 15 Pisces-Virgo was square to Rodger's Mars at 14 Gemini! Hammerstein's words were brought to life, animated, by Rodger's music. Again, quite a creatively tense and powerful bond, with one nodal contact complementing the other, i.e., Saturn and Mars—the bond that helped this team create the historic musicals *Oklahoma, Carousel, South Pacific*, and *The King and I*.

A lovely example is seen between Princess Grace (November 12, 1929) and Prince Ranier of Monaco (October 31, 1923). This was the fairy-tale love bond: European prince and Philadelphia beauty off in their private kingdom. This was love felt and espied across a crowded room, this was "getting to node you" in classic romantic fashion: Princess Grace had her Nodal Axis in 11 Taurus-Scorpio 34 precisely conjunct Prince Ranier's Venus and Jupiter [*both*] at 11 Taurus 34 and 11 Scorpio 02, respectively! Additionally, her Jupiter at 14 Gemini was square *his* Nodal Axis at 16 Virgo-Pisces!

The cases can go on and on: President George Bush (June 12, 1924) and "out-of-nowhere" Vice-Presidential candidate Dan Quayle (February 4, 1947) were clearly brought together by reciprocal Nodal contacts and more; Bill Clinton (August 19, 1946) has his Sun at 26 Leo, mighty and proud, and Hillary Clinton (October 26, 1947) has her Nodal Axis at 24 Taurus-Scorpio, tightly square his Sun. That is his hook-up to the synthesis of her strengths; that is the bond of tolerance for her in the midst of the stress from all her husband's misadventures. We could surmise as well that his charismatic way to success fronts for her deepest professional dreams for herself.

Chart 8: Martin/Lewis, Double-Ring Horoscope

A final example (chart 8, p. 58): certainly one of the great comedy teams of the last century, Dean Martin (June 7, 1917 at 11:55 P.M. in Steubenville, Ohio) and Jerry Lewis (March 16, 1926 at 12:15 P.M. in Newark, New Jersey).

Jerry's Sun-Uranus conjunction in Pisces squares Dean's Midheaven, his Neptune square's Dean's Mercury, his Saturn squares Dean's Uranus, and the Lewis Mars in Capricorn conjoins Martin's Moon and opposes his Saturn. But above all—with these measurements already showing the powerful Lewis driving the performing relationship—*there is Jerry's Pluto conjunct Dean's Nodal Axis, and Dean's Moon conjunct Jerry's Nodal Axis!!*

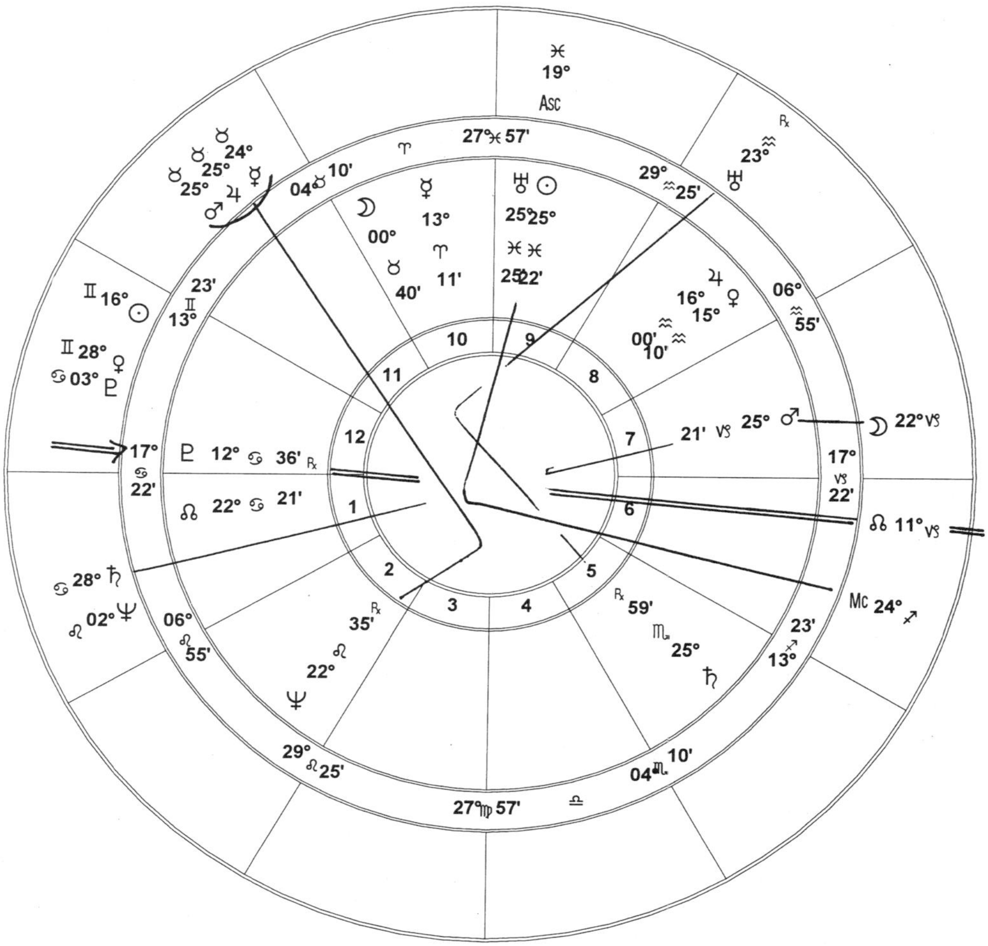

Chart 8

Inner Chart
Jerry Lewis
Mar. 16, 1926, 12:15 P.M. EST
Newark, New Jersey
74W10, 40N44

Outer Chart
Dean Martin
June 7, 1917, 11:55 P.M. CST
Steubenville, Ohio
80W37, 40N22

Happy Relationships

This couple has been married forty-four years. He is airplane-pilot craggy-handsome and she is conservative-showgirl beautiful. Both are in fine physical shape, retired, affluent. They are together constantly and seem not to have a care in the world. They have long been through the early career development stress, the income-building tensions, the job fears, the responsibilities of children, and they have faced everything together with great success and fulfillment.

I asked them if they had ever thought or said that their marriage "was made in heaven," or that each was clearly soul mate to the other. "Rick" replied, "No . . . but I can say we have never had an argument. Sure we've discussed things strongly with each other, but never an argument."

I suggested to them that they clearly were fulfilling each other's needs, and that gain and loss balance had been achieved easily from the very beginning of their relationship. They agreed instantly.

Let's look at those needs individually first, and then together synastrically.

Chart 9: "Rick"

"Rick" is sixty-nine in 2000. His Sun-Moon blend in Aquarius, reinforced strongly by Mars, projects "humanistic energies administered to the public through the intellect and through the sense of bureaucratic expediency (p. 60). These are the positions of a public leader: the rugged individual campaigner who sways the crowd and makes things happen." Rick fits this description precisely: for his entire career he was a high-profile lobbyist, primarily in Washington, D.C., active in the management of legislation for the country. As part of his job, he was constantly active socially.

He is a man of careful thought, deliberate thought, and rigid routine (Saturn conjunct Mercury), who has been very successful with these faculties (Mercury=Jupiter/Pluto). Rick and his wife happily live a precise schedule, with each day's activities mirroring the day before.

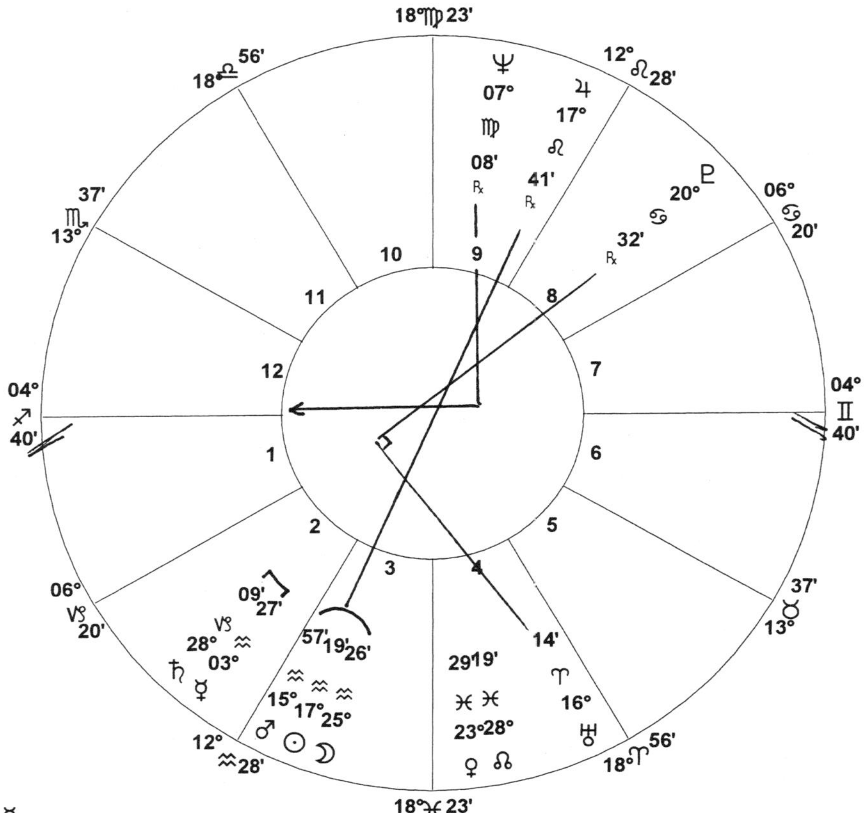

☿ = ♃/♇

	☽	☉	☿	♀	♂	♃	♄	♅	♆	♇	☊	Mc
☉	∥											
☿												
♀												
♂		☌s 01°23										
♃	#	☍a # 00°22	q s 00°46		☍a # 01°44							
♄			☌s ∥ 05°18									
♅		⚹s 01°05	Qa 00°47		⚹a 00°17	△a 01°27						
♆				q s 01°21								
♇				△s 02°57				□a 04°18	∠a 01°36			
☊				☌a 04°49			⚹a 00°10					
Mc		⊼s 01°04	⚼a 00°04	☍a 05°06	⊼s 02°26			⊼s 02°09		⚹a 02°09		
Asc		Qa 00°40	⚹s ∥ 01°13		Qs 00°43		∥		□a 02°29	⚼a 00°53		

Chart 9

“Rick”

In the time of knowing Rick, what emerges through this strong demeanor is a warm aesthetic sense as well: music, cinema, reading, learning, all of which he discusses with lights in his eyes (Venus in Pisces quindecile Neptune, trine Pluto).

The Pluto-Uranus square is a subgeneration signature and simply does not seem to apply here in Rick's life significantly, except that he prides himself on knowing as much as he can possibly learn (Uranus rules the 3rd), and he is very uncomfortable with (Pluto rules the 12th) the unknown. The entire focus of Rick's profile is social activity and deliberated persuasion for the public good, the grace of aesthetics, and the record of and continuing interest in sports (Sagittarius Ascendant; Jupiter opposes Mars, ruler of the 5th), children, and knowledge.

His needs are very clear: the reigning need is to be effective in social and promotional administration of ideas for the common good (it bears repeating that he appreciates information and intelligence enormously)—note Mars oriental, the energies, selling a cause—and the adherence to a *rigid* routine of day-to-day behavior. *Rick's mate will need to need what Rick offers in order for Rick to be fulfilled in the relationship.*

Chart 10: "Jennifer"

"Jennifer" has an intense focus in Taurus with the Moon in Capricorn (p. 62). There should be a strong desire here for influence; she has the need to make things happen . . . or perhaps to be with a mate who makes things happen. There is a strain of idealism here (Sun with Mercury, intensified by Uranus), *correctness*, but the complex is opposed by Mars *retrograde, in Libra*, and the triple conjunction is in the 12th House. Jennifer probably will not be able to get the job done herself, so she will be relying on her mate to achieve her potentials for her, with her. In other words, they must see eye-to-eye about this, where they can go *together* to be fulfilled in growth individually.

Note that in the Sun-Uranus-Mercury opposition with Mars, that axis is squared by the Moon and it takes place in Cadent Houses, with the Moon ruling the 3rd. Here we can anticipate *reaction rather than instigation.* As our

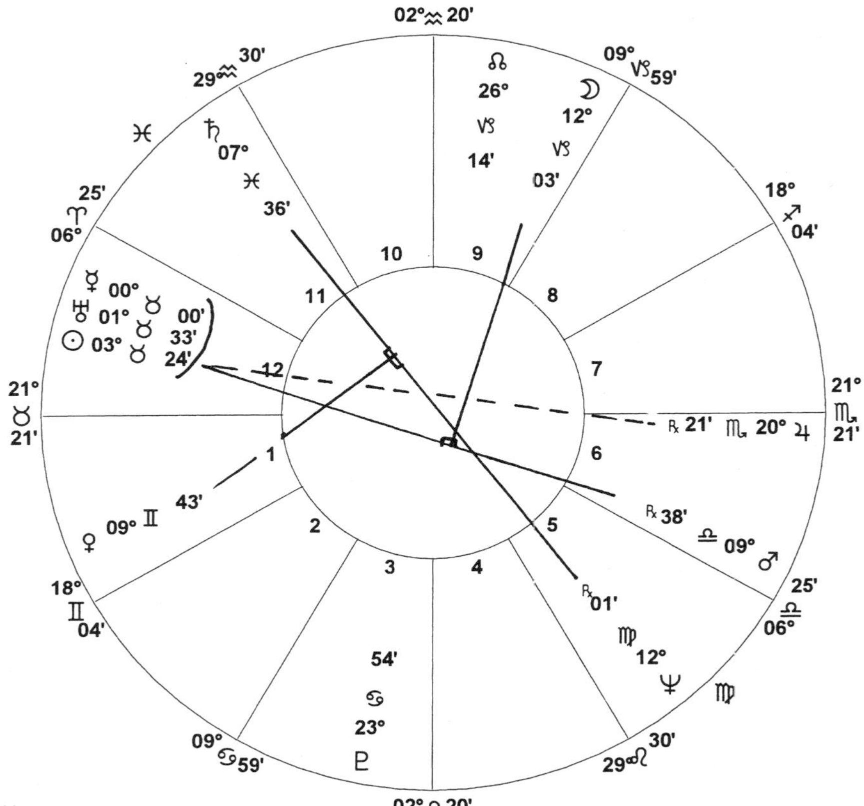

	☽	☉	☿	♀	♂	♃	♄	♅	♆	♇	☊	Mc
☉												
☿		☌a 03°24										
♀	⊼s ǂ 02°19											
♂	□s 02°25			△s 00°06								
♃		q a 01°57										
♄			ǂ	□s 02°08	⊼a 02°02							
♅		☌s 01°51	☌a ∥ 01°32									
♆	△s 00°01			□a 02°18			☍a 04°26					
♇	ǂ			∠s ∥ 00°50		△s 03°33	⚼a 01°18					
☊			□s 03°46	⚼a 01°31				□s 05°18	⚼s 00°47	☍a 02°20		
Mc		□a 01°04	□s 02°20			Qa 00°01		□s 00°48			☌s 06°06	
Asc						☍s 01°00	Qs 01°45			⚹a 02°33	△a 04°53	

Chart 10

"Jennifer"

first impression of the horoscope forms itself, we see so much fitting into the Mars-in-Libra image.

Saturn is in the 11th signifying an enormous need for love. Saturn rules the 9th and is opposed by Neptune, suggesting strongly that Jennifer's education did not continue into college. Venus square to this axis, Venus ruling the Ascendant, suggests early home development issues (as does Uranus conjunct the Sun, rulers of the 10th and 4th, respectively). Jennifer was a show dancer, beauty contest winner, and a busy model in her late teenage years, but all this stopped when she met Rick and married.

The picture shows a dependency upon the mate (mirroring the Pluto sextile the Ascendant). This is conclusively stated by Jupiter, ruler of the 8th (the mate's resources) quindecile to the Sun, and Jupiter is trine Pluto, ruler of the 7th.

Jennifer needs to ally herself to someone else's structure that will be strong, successful, and beautiful for her. She needs much love, and these gains will attract a tremendous idealized loyalty and supportive compliance from her.

Neither Rick nor Jennifer shows any tension at all related to the 7th House, except perhaps for the wide Saturn conjunction with Rick's Mercury which does rule his 7th House. I do not see this as a signal of a loss situation with regard to his relationship with Jennifer (perhaps with others in his life), *because his Saturn-Mercury conjunction is what she needs*—and, as we shall see immediately below, the conjunction is what her Nodal Axis, Sun-Uranus-and Mercury conjunction, and Midheaven *all* tie into!

There is much more here, but our discussion clarifies easily that these two people portray a high potential of fitting each other perfectly. Let's see their horoscopes together:

Chart 11: Rick and Jennifer Double-Ringed Horoscope

Immediately (p. 64), we see that Rick's powerful sober thought and rigid demeanor position of **Saturn conjunct Mercury is conjunct Jennifer's Nodal Axis.** Dare we say—but surely we can begin to feel—that these two

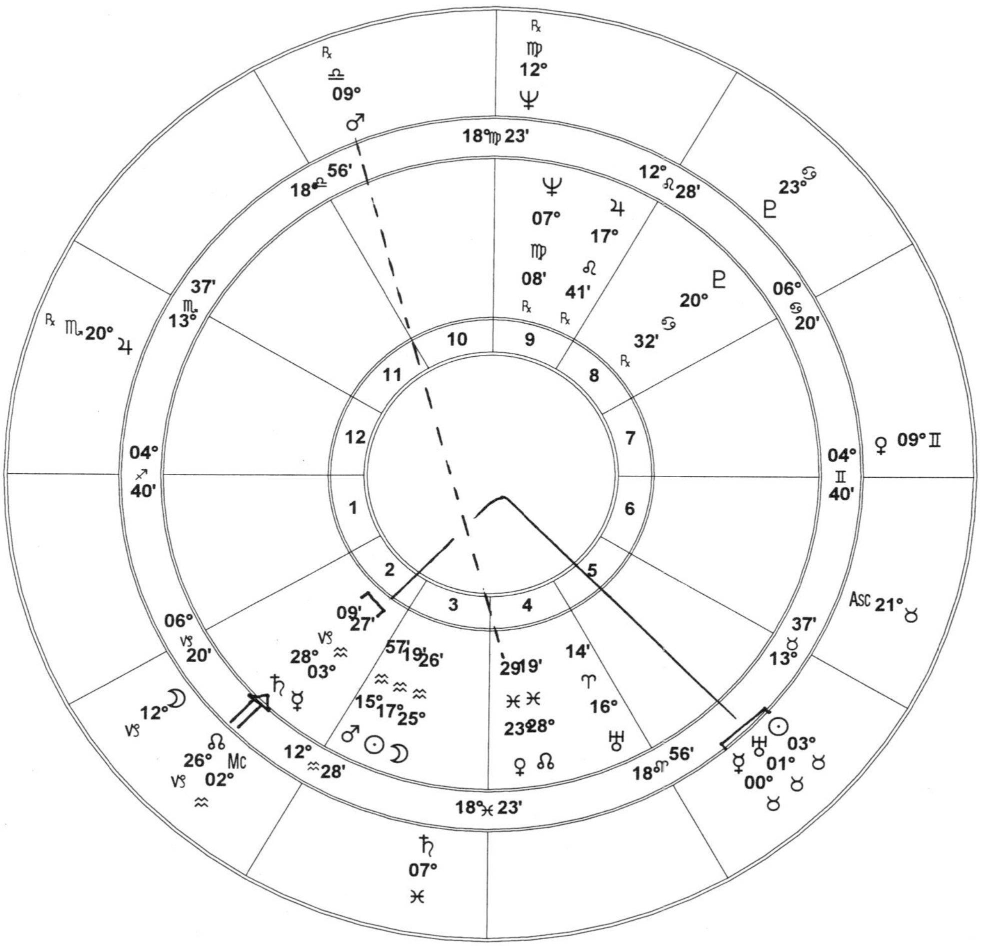

Chart 11

Inner Chart
"Rick"

Outer Chart
"Jennifer"

people have been together before? These positions are also tightly squared by Jennifer's Sun-Uranus-Mercury triple conjunction! This tells us that Rick administers so much of life organization and thinking for Jennifer. There may be tension with this dominant personality trait in Rick's *other* relationships, but not with her. From her perspective, his Saturn-Mercury squares her Sun-Uranus-Mercury and conjoins her Nodal Axis: somehow it is felt/meant to be that his strong thought demeanor leads her way. There is no question about it.

Her Mars$_{Rx}$ in Libra is quindecile his very sensitive Venus: here is the aesthetic, sexual bond, and, as well, her tacit support and grace with his strongly routinized ways. Jennifer is indeed beautiful—they both are—and this immediately sets them apart when they walk into a room. There is no doubt that Rick needs that image and honors that reality. She basks in it.

Her Ascendant trines his Midheaven, another statement of her living her life through his, through his status, his career receiving her complete support. Remember: these people were born in the early 1930s, inheriting the socially prescribed gender roles from their parents and their society at that time. Rick is the breadwinner; Jennifer is the beautiful housewife and mother.

Is this how they related before? Did they find each other again?

These people are utterly delightful, appear completely at peace in their intimacy with one another, and we are grateful to them for sharing their portraits.

Technical Synastric Considerations

In synastric measurement technique, it is practicable to relate a natal planet or point in one person's horoscope *to a natal Midpoint measurement in a second person's horoscope*, using the 90-degree Midpoint Sort [please see pages 303–333 in *Synthesis & Counseling in Astrology*].

For Jennifer and Rick, the synthesis picture of compatibility is reinforced strongly:

- **Her Moon=his Sun/Asc, Jupiter/Asc:** feelings and needs are all-important in relationship; kindness, largesse, happiness.
- **Her Node=his MC/Asc:** pleasantness, social contacts are easy.
- **Her Venus=his Mercury/Uranus:** his imaging of love, spontaneous recognition, and arousal.
- **Her Asc=his Sun/Moon (!):** [21Taurus21 to 21Aquarius23] Greatest fit, openness, security, high-focus importance in partnership terms.
- **His Sun-Mars-Jupiter=her Neptune/Pluto:** magnetism, in love with love, at one with the way things should be.
- **His Venus=her Node/Asc:** Pleasantness, affectionate associations.
- **His MC=her Sun/MC:** [In synastry, duplication on either side of the equation is acceptable since a different person is involved.] His career and social status afford her ego recognition, success, fulfillment; their achieving together and getting what the relationship deserves.

3

FEAR AND DISILLUSIONMENT

Expressions of Animus and Anima

In my university days, the theoretical frameworks for the psyche developed by Freud and Jung were differentiated from each other in two ways. First: Freud was for people growing up, which captured the instinctive hedonistic press into life of the Freudian orientation, while Jung was for people over thirty-five, which captured the thinking-person's orientation to primal meanings within life. The second generalized but not unreasonable distinction was that Freud approached life development from a particularly male orientation, while Jung differentiated between the psychology of men and the psychology of women.

Theorists developing ideas and applications upon the Jungian base present the gender-differentiation theme with fundamental reference and orientation to Adam and Eve, to Eve conceived *out of* Adam. Adam contained the God spirit ("Made in the likeness of God"). Eve was within Adam. Eve issued forth containing the God spirit *and* containing Adam, within *her*. The bi-gender orientation of man and woman is a clear metaphor and it is invested with primal creative purpose: *the woman is within the man; the man is within the woman.*

The human being's androgynous nature is personified, preserved, and taught throughout mythologies in all cultures. Polarities of reference and judgment emerge from this orientation: there are the Yang and Yin, light and dark, good and evil, pleasure and pain. But the integrating concept necessary for the appreciation of life is that *these polarities work together holistically;* one pole requires the other, just as silence defines sound, as sound defines silence; as I is defined by Thou, the dynamic of personal growth through relationship.

Jung labeled the masculine component within the female the *animus* and the female component within the male the *anima*.[22] These concepts are *archetypes* because they are typical of the human condition, they are primal, they are existentially fundamental.

One part of our understanding of the animus/anima construct is that the animus in the woman and the anima in the man help each gender to understand the other. The animus offers the female an empathic understanding of the hard, guarded, driving, and critical part of being male. The anima offers the male empathic understanding of the soft, sensitive, expressive, and moody part of being female. Again we see the polarities of behaviors established for the male and female archetypes in society. As we have seen, these male/female expectations are put upon us by our culture, and we must traffic through the labeling and overlays of conditioning to be ourselves. The animus/anima balancing works to help us do this in our relationships.

A second part of our understanding is that, because of the archetypal societal conditioning, **we *project* animus/anima constructs upon people with whom we relate.** In relating to the woman, the man projects upon her his anima construct within himself. In relating to the man, the woman projects upon him her animus construct formed within her. "He/She is just perfect!" means "he/she is just what I want for myself." This is the opinion we reach

---

22 The two Latin words are derived from the Latin *animare*, the infinitive "to give life to, to animate." The "-a" is the feminine ending; the "-us" is the masculine ending. Sometimes the translation is given as "spirit."

upon successful projection. The other person is precisely what we need for completion, for reflection of Self, for unity, for wholeness.[23]

This is what "being in love" means: a man and a woman project their positive images onto each other at the same time. This is the elusive perfection of relationship, and in chapter 4 we will have more to say about love.

The idealized projections come from our acculturation process, our sociometric level of social development. The images are preached to us by everyone around us, and to one degree or another of success or failure they are modeled for us by our parents. We internalize how we "should be" as male or female, and we begin to project *how the other gender "should be" for us in relationship*. We say, "If I were a man/woman, boy! I would be. . . ." or, "The man/woman I want will be. . . ."

At the same time, our individual horoscope is speaking out also, through our individualized organization of needs. Our inner environment is meeting the external environment, *the animus/anima constructs are being formed in relation to our individual needs as well as in relation to societal imprint*; the search for relationship is started, and, within this complex process, complications begin.

But how long does the idealized, projected animus/anima image last? Our language offers many clichés (truisms) about the bubble bursting, about someone turning out not to be what we thought he or she was, someone not being what he or she was "cracked up to be," about our being let down, deceived, our making a big, big mistake. The animus/anima projections that issue from our unconscious cannot cope with the rigors of reality: fantasy and realism have great difficulty mixing. *The challenges and stress of everyday life burst the creatively conceived bubble of projection.*

In the awakening of disappointment, in the crisis of rejection, in the slight of being ignored, the animus and anima become negative; they implode and then lash out. Since the idealized construct has been let down, the anima in

---

23 See Sanford, 17–19, 59: "Whenever a man or woman fascinates us we can be sure that a projected content of the unconscious is at work. In their all-too-human reality people are not fascinating; it is the archetypal figures of the unconscious that are fascinating."

the man turns inward, moods follow, then self-deprecation (feminine archetypal disposition); the sensitive part of Self is subjected to feelings of pain, a kind of emotional hysteria can form. To discharge this pain, the negative anima then explodes outward in emotionally rationalized criticism, prima donna posturing about perpetual hurts; and, with the projection of altogether negative feelings, tyranny of the targeted woman. In turn, to the woman, the anima-possessed man appears like a weak, melodramatic, emotional misfit.

The animus in the woman turns inward with self-deprecation and feelings of worthlessness, followed by enormous disappointment and loneliness; thought processes go nowhere, opinions become irrational. To discharge this pain, the negative animus then can explode outward in emotional criticism, illogical extremism, and rejection. Here in defensive mode, often in camouflage of what really is at the core of upset, the projected negative feelings tyrannize the man with criticism, devaluation, and threatened rejection (masculine archetypal disposition). In turn, to the man, the woman becomes an intolerable shrew.

The interreactions between man and woman under reality conditions—between hurt anima and aroused animus, respectively—are hurtful and ugly, and yet they can eventually lead to realism, to refinement, to balance, mutual respect, trust . . . and intimacy. This process must be consciously worked through with an effort to know oneself and respect that same maturing effort in others.

As we begin to discuss some negative animus/anima projections, each of us all too vividly will meet up with parts of ourselves in the descriptions. Such study—more strongly developed than we are doing in this book—is impressively presented in many specialist texts dealing with Jungian analysis, available in bookstore psychology and self-help departments. One of the most accessible and helpful is the superb volume *The Invisible Partners* by John Sanford, noted in the bibliography.

It is important here to mention emotional honesty because, under negative animus/anima projection, emotional honesty can quickly disappear. Emotional hurt (upset anima) and vitriolic anger (upset animus) exceed reason and depart from the rational. Past hurts are brought out from psychic storage and are re-inflicted onto present newly hurt sensibilities. Long strings of accusations stream out and create branch upon branch of argument. In turn, these amassed hurts are stored up once again, only to be revived during the next round of confrontation.

It sounds so simple to realize that what has actually happened is that the idealized projections are discovered to have been unrealistic in the first place. Yet this is the natural process of acculturation and relating! We desperately *want* to be completed somehow, to find out-there the complement to what is in-here. The I searches for the Thou in grand, fantasy-formed dimension. We project this model onto a person-screen, someone who will reflect our projection back to us. We need it greatly, we project it powerfully. It is a projection that is enigmatically created to fail.

As we shall see, it is *knowing the process of what is transpiring* that can settle things down and free us from the tyranny of the idealized.

The anima can be seen as active wherever emotions are at work in a man. Everything is intensified, exaggerated, and it is all stored up. How easy is it for most men to express their feelings? The emotionally expressive male does not fit the male archetype of our society.

Sanford says, "A man who always avoids emotionally toned encounters with other people is contained [unconsciously focused] within the Mother. One way for him to get out of his Mother complex is to express himself in relationship. If he fails to do so he remains emotionally a little boy who is afraid of women, who resents them if they don't keep him happy, and who is out of touch with his own masculine strength."[24]

This is only reasonable. How many men "marry their mother," or, at least, marry a part of their mother in someone else. This dimension of the mother

---

24 Sanford, 37–38.

is desperately needed—that need is routined—and *must be* a trait in the significant other. The relationship then becomes an opportunity for seeing to unfinished business from childhood, to preserving security with someone who probably made all the emotional decisions for the boy (man) and must continue to do so.

So, when we see a pronounced mother-influence measurement construct in a male's horoscope [any planet or point conjunct or square the Lunar Nodal axis (2.5-degree orb), Pluto square conjunct or opposed the Moon, or possibly other hard aspects to the Moon, usually accompanied by a hard aspect to a significator of the parental axis], we must appreciate the potential of anima formation and projection *in the guise of the maternal image and its influence*. This projection is designed to echo the mother relationship . . . or to avoid it completely. In the former case, the man perpetuates the past relationship; in the latter possibility, he appears to rescue himself from the past relationship, but this is rarely successful without full understanding of the process that is transpiring.

It is easily understandable that a man on the receiving end of a negative animus onslaught from his female partner will interpret the onslaught as demeaning and critical and will fear rejection. There is a reversion to the small boy within him. He will be painfully hurt. Then his anima—terribly disappointed—becomes negative, gets turned around, and implodes in deep frustration, moodiness, and noncommunicative sorrow. His mind plays out scenarios of freeing himself—sometimes to an extreme—and these scenarios create guilt. Depression begins to deepen. His Moon and Venus are jeopardized. Intimacy, sexuality, and relationship, of course, become/appear impossible.

Sanford observes, "The anima not only interferes with a man's emotional reactions, she can interfere with his thinking as well. For instance, when a man is anima-possessed [in defense against the fear of rejection] he may begin to give forth *opinions* instead of genuine thinking [the latter, being the masculine prerogative]. It is as though the anima begins to talk right through him [in retaliation], and she [the anima] expresses herself as though she had an animus, which means that she expresses opinions without regard to facts, relationship, or logic. When a man is in this state of mind he begins to argue in a peevish way, and his masculine objectivity is quite lost in a sea of emotionally toned and irrational opinions that prove resistant to reasonable discussion."[25]

In short, the projected anima has broken down. The fascination, the initial beguilement, is gone, ripped down by day-to-day routine and realistic perspective. Unless the man knows what is going on, he suffers terribly from disillusionment; the bubble has burst, the mistake has been made, what will his family think, etc.

Within this drama, the woman inflicting the negative animus is instinctively doing it to defend herself. Her Sun and Mars are strongly aroused. Is she turning the tables within her disappointment about something in the man's makeup? Is she becoming a stern disapproving, nonsupporting father? Is she acting out how her father behaved or how she imagined him behaving through her own collapsed self-worth filter? Is she destroying the man before she herself is pilloried? After all, her partner has not expressed, communicated any compliments, affection, love to her for the longest time. What does this mean? What is his moodiness about?

Children get caught within the parental drama all the time. How can a child feel attended to, let alone loved, by a mother in a strong, self-absorbed animus opinionation onslaught, or by a father in a self-absorbed anima withdrawal orientation. Where is the anima expression of care and emotions in the mother and father; where is the animus expression of leadership and confidence in each of the parents? Sanford points out that this situation is exacerbated when *the father has relinquished the masculine role of disciplinarian [leader] and forced the mother to assume this role [animus] in the family.* And here we see vividly part of the Saturn-retrograde phenomenon, with the mother's influence becoming paramount by default, when the parents' relationship with the child is out of balance.

---

25 Sanford, 41.

It is clear that the male and the female fear criticism, rejection, and abandonment by the other; this is what is behind the fear of intimacy, getting too close with/to our vulnerabilities. It is clear that personal vulnerabilities inhibit exposure of one's Self to another because such exposure will reveal the burst bubble, the breakdown of the idealized projection each had for the other. Relationship then becomes a battle, to one degree or another. Individual needs defensively adjust thresholds of tolerance for the other's failures. Routine sets in and the modeling process for the children is set.

Rescue

A man assailed by negative animus behavior from the female partner must realize first that what he is hearing is irrational, that it comes from some source that almost always is somewhere else rather than within him—he is the scapegoat. Second, he must try as hard as he can to respond within his own masculine image. Jungian literature recommends simple statements like, "What is really bothering you? How can I help with this?"

And counselors caution that enough inquiry is enough. Efforts to salvage the situation must then be left to the suffering female. The man has made his offer to help, and that's that . . . until the next appropriate time for the offer of discussion/help.

The woman who realizes that she is in the throes (possessed state) of a negative animus projection must ask herself, "Where have I been disappointed or hurt in my feelings and have not come to grips with it?" Remember, it may have been the man's negative anima implosion, self-absorption, moodiness about something entirely away from the woman that triggered within her *her* fears of criticism, rejection, abandonment. What if, at the first sign of upset in her partner, his moodiness/withdrawal, she had asked, "You seem hurt. What should we talk about to help this out?" At the very least, she would have reasonably absolved herself from complicity. The partner would have been given the opportunity to talk it out; if the cause of his concern were she, he could easily have presented his case **in a discussion situation that was**

clearly *not* threatened by the negative-animus backlash from his partner. He had nothing to fear.

And this is the key point for growth, maturation, empathy, and the support of intimacy: **to be able to express feelings, show vulnerability one to another, without fear of criticism, rejection, or abandonment.**

For example, Sanford says that *if a man is emotionally expressive in his relationship, he will not fall into moods.* This emotional expressivity rescues him from "the clutches of his anima." If a woman feels strong and decisive within her identity without having to prove it to herself and others, she will not need to rage and criticize in negative animus fashion. *Her confidence within her role as a woman and as an individual rescues her from the clutches of her animus.*

These rescuing realisms are commonsensical. The bubble is adjusted. *Respect for being human enters the picture and actually displaces the disappointment for not being ideal.*

The problems challenging relationship are practically everywhere. Overstated criticism about table manners, management of clothes ready for the laundry, or how one is dressed to go out to dinner may be the catalyst for upset, the outlet for disillusionment felt in other, far more personal and serious departments of life. What if, after a relationship develops, it is revealed that the man or the woman (or both) shows some sexual dysfunction, something less than the ideal that was projected by each upon the other, or was initially overlooked in the exciting effort to establish a relationship?

Perhaps the man has a small penis, which the woman begins to realize is not suited to her aesthetic or sensory ideal built up over years of fantasy and experience. Perhaps the man's job stress and perhaps the extra drinks he uses to calm down at night make his erections less than strong, his desire less frequent with time. Perhaps he is projecting on to her his anxiety about his sexual performance, blaming her in the subtlest of ways. The woman's animus can be aroused in defense; the criticisms delivered devastatingly, almost certainly camouflaged within some other argument like helping around the house, going out more, breaking routine, taking a vacation.

What if it is revealed that the woman is nonorgasmic in relationship with him, having heretofore camouflaged the lack of response? What if she hears him now talking about sexual attributes she does not have? What if it emerges that she has lost interest in their routined schedule and scenario for sex? She never initiates sex any more. The man easily suffers here, the disappointment weakening his anima. The moodiness and withdrawal follow. The distance between the man and woman grows.

What if the man develops prostate cancer after twenty years of marriage—a marriage that seemed to have gotten adjusted within all the cross-pressures—and, as a result, even with modern medicine and techniques, becomes impotent (perhaps actually rescuing him finally from "sexual responsibility"!)? What if the woman undergoes a radical mastectomy? What has happened to their individual self-image and the projected image of each to the other?

Because of sexual considerations, each person has become *eminently more vulnerable* than he/she was earlier in the relationship. Fears return and come closer and closer to the core of Self. Old pains come out of storage. Resurrected bitterness displaces the heretofore fragilely engineered trust.

Yet, even in these instances—with psycho-neurological sexual problems—*understanding the process of communicating to each other without the fears of criticism, rejection, abandonment can create a stronger bond in relationship.* This is possible through self-understanding first; then honesty; then confidence; and finally, respect for the same process in the partner.

A client of mine telephoned yesterday. She is extremely cerebral. She is living in her second marriage, to a man twenty-three years her senior. *Her Saturn rules her 7th* and is opposed by Mars in Virgo (you can immediately feel her animus as master of detail and technique). This axis is squared by the Sun and Moon in Gemini. The axis falls in the 3rd–9th House polarity of mindset and reaction.

During her early development, my client received "only criticism from her father . . . he was never satisfied." Her Moon and Venus (anima symbols) are conjunct in the 12th (you can immediately feel her anima as withdrawn, patterned after the mother), and her mother was very protective of her—perhaps they protected each other from the father.

The call came in for an update because June's husband was away on a business trip, he was cheating on her, she had found him out by snooping here and there; she had hired a detective to follow him, and, when he was to return, she planned quite a confrontation [Tr Saturn, ruler of the 7th, close to conjoining the Sun; SA Saturn=Sun applying within one degree]. As June told me this, I heard the hurt animus speaking within her and preparing its vengeance. The bubble had burst. Her confidence was gone.

In discussing the situation further, I asked about their sex life in the recent time. She said it had been "horrible" *since her baby was born three years ago*. She had been troubled by depression throughout her life—all keyed to the early home experiences, in my opinion and with her agreement. And indeed, the depression had reappeared postpartum for the past three years, tying it to the birth of the child.

Was her husband dissatisfied? What had now happened to *his* anima? Had she asked him about his feelings? Was he emotionally solicitous about *her* feelings? Was there any communication about these things? Had each grown afraid of the other? How was she explaining his philandering to her over-busy mind? Just imagine how—now not working at a job and staying at home for the third year with the baby—how idleness had brought so much cerebral over-analysis to these questions and *revived her early family history*. Now, the fears of criticism, rejection, and abandonment were enormous. The disillusioned animus was awakened in defense.

An Astrological Look

The entire process of animus/anima formation and their balancing within reality experience is dedicated to improving relationship. The presumption is that we first learn to relate with ourselves, to diminish the distance between us and ourselves; that's where the conflicts begin, and those conflicts are projected onto others.

Relationship works toward wholeness. Complementation. Mutual support. The I is completed by the Thou. We *do* need others to reflect to us, to show us who *we* are. Ideally, with this reflection and knowledge, we find the meaning in and the enjoyment of being alive.

Swiss astrologers Hajo Banzhaf and Brigitte Theler have done substantive work with the animus/anima construct and have offered an astrological hypothesis linking these two Jungian archetypes to the synastric balance and complementation of the astrological Elements: Fire, Air, Earth, and Water.[26]

Banzhaf and Theler work with the acknowledged Sun and Mars reference to the animus and the Moon and Venus reference to the anima, and they postulate that becoming related (loving) "appears to be the longing of our soul for wholeness that drives [us] to connect with what we lack." *What we lac*k is keyed in the horoscope by the lack of accent of one of the Elements.[27]

This is quite reasonable: if the male sees the female as "everything I need," she is supplying *something he lacks*. If he has no accentuation of Fire in his horoscope (with Sun, Moon, Mercury, Venus, Mars, Jupiter, and Saturn positioned in other Elements), he *needs* Fire. He meets someone strongly Fire-emphasized, and his anima projection is fulfilled by the fiery personality, the enlivened life, the exciting motivation and daring.

Banzhaf and Theler say, "As long as even one element remains more or less unconscious and is lacking in our consciousness, we perceive reality in a distorted and incomplete manner. . . . During the course of life, the missing element increasingly becomes an important topic, since we not only lack it in terms of our wholeness, but also because it is frequently the source of our errors."[28]

---

26 Please see Banzhaf and Theler, *Secrets of Love & Partnership*, noted in the bibliography.

27 Banzhaf and Theler do not count Uranus, Neptune, Pluto (because they move slowly and are generational in reference), Ascendant, and Midheaven (because they are not planets) in their Element count.

28 Banzhaf and Theler, 4.

We tend to link up with a person who complements us by ***corresponding to our missing Element.*** This sense of not actually *embodying* the missing Element is important here: when the anima or animus projection of idealized perfection is made by the man/woman, the bubble is set to burst in time (its extremism concocted by the unconscious dooms it to unfulfillment or failure); it is unreasonable to expect perfect, complete embodiment of our "inner searching image." The best we can do is welcome into our life the person who corresponds to our lack, who provides much of it to make us whole. *This caution of understanding here in our discussion is the realism that must prevail to balance anima/animus constructs within relationship and set the stage for intimacy.*

Astrologer Erin Sullivan writes in the same direction, "A lack of Earth will attract Earth to it, lack of Air accretes Airy types, on through the elements of Fire and Water. When we lack an element, the deeper self will seek it out and find it in others so that we may have the benefit of it in our immediate environment. Speaking more psychologically, if we have an undeveloped or sleeping characteristic, it is very frequently projected on to others who will collude in this projection and live it out for us."[29]

Look once again at the happy couple's horoscopes (charts 9 and 10) on pp. 60 and 62.

Jennifer has no statement in the Fire Element. Basically, this suggests a low level of motivation, temperament, daring, passion, courage on her own. For Jennifer, her animus projection must include *a specification for Fire*, for the Element to be made up, for someone to supply her with leadership, excited spontaneity, force.

Her husband of forty-four years, Rick has one statement in Fire, Jupiter in Leo [the Uranus position and the Ascendant position are not included in this judgement initially; see footnote 6]. Here follows part of perhaps the finest description of Jupiter in Leo I have ever studied:

---

29 Sullivan, p. 141.

> . . . an awareness of social position can stimulate the ambition to be the best-dressed, most esteemed, or most envied member of a particular group. There may be a desire to own more living space, jewels, or worldly goods than any one person needs, not so much for the sake of security, but for sheer ostentation.
>
> Conscientious people of this temperament will use their organizational abilities to serve others less fortunate than themselves . . . a sense of *noblesse oblige*.
>
> This combination is propitious for executive work, especially in government service or in large, well-established enterprises.[30]

The description not only fits Rick perfectly *but his wife as well,* i.e., he has complemented her where she had a conspicuous lack. I shared lunch with this couple just an hour ago, and without any prompting at all from me, Jennifer said twice in fun and truth, "I do whatever he tells me to do, don't I dear?" Here is her recognition of his Fire complement.

Rick was involved for his entire career with legislative lobbying among state and federal governments for major corporations. He tells expense-account tales, he has owned eighteen different cars, now a top-of-the-line Mercedes and a red Corvette convertible, and his wife is a fashion plate and wears the largest diamond ring I have ever seen outside of a museum.

Dean Martin, the great singer and comedian partner with Jerry Lewis (see chart 8, p. 58), had no Fire statement in his horoscope. Recall Martin's lackadaisical, easy-going image.

Jerry Lewis supplied the intense motivation, daring, and strategic thrust to the historic comedy team. Jerry conducted all the business for the duo while Dean played golf. *Jerry Lewis' Mercury is in Aries, linked with Martin's Nodal axis.*

> Mercury in Aries describes a person who is quick and impulsive in speech and thought. He tends to be a glib talker who enunciates his ideas with an animated expression accompanied by sweeping ges-

---

30 Moore and Douglas, 108.

> tures of the hands . . . an incendiary brightness as the mind spins like a pinwheel casting off dazzling showers of sparks.[31]

Here again is perfect complementation.

Fascinatingly, Hitler's horoscope has no accentuation in Water (an enormous difficulty orientating to emotional values, therefore a projection to grand references beyond interpersonal relationships, like religion or the fantastic). His mate Eva Braun (see p. 55), while tied with Hitler through the incredible Nodal Axis and other synastric measurements, did not have any accentuation in Water either. Was there really an emotional orientated complementation between them? How intimate could that relationship have become? *Were they both lost in the same arena?*

Prince Ranier's birth date (see p. 57) shows all Water and Air, *no Fire or Earth.* The incredible relationship with Grace Kelly is suggested through Fire fulfillment (a glowing, anchored, dignified, practical persistence) of his lack (characteristic moody, lonely, withdrawn, impractical softness).

Banzhaf and Theler study as well how a man or woman may react to the idealized other who provides the missing Element, *after the bubble has inevitably burst*, in terms of the person's animus (Sun, Mars in the woman) or anima (the Moon, Venus in the male).[32] Basically the thesis is that—for example—if we lack Fire and our planets *of the opposite gender* (Sun, Mars in the female; Moon, Venus in the male) are in Earth, we will start to complain that the other person is *not* as down to earth (Earth), cool and inventive (Air), or imaginative and sensitive (Water) as would correspond to our inner image projected upon him or her. This is not difficult to understand: we will complain about an underachievement in terms of Element(s) projected from our animus or anima planets.

So, if we lack Earth, and our planets of the opposite gender are located in Fire, Air, or Water, we will start to complain that he or she is *not* as spontaneous

---

31 Moore and Douglas, 62–63.

32 Banzhaf and Theler, 32.

(Fire), smart or clever (Air), or as tactful and devoted (Water) as would correspond to our inner image projected upon him or her.

But, here I feel the thesis becomes perhaps oversystematized. It can become complicated, especially in the man's case as the projection of the anima, involving the Moon, is involving as well, psychodynamically, the symbol of his reigning need. And how do we portion out the projections issuing from the Moon (or Sun) or Venus (or Mars), which most frequently are in different Signs, different Elements.

I have personally resolved this by knowing the supreme relevance of the Sun-Moon blend within the individual's horoscope, and knowing that, in every horoscope, *one of the luminaries is dramatically part of the individual animus or anima projection as well.* Then, in fulfillment of the Sun-Moon blend, we are learning about the dimensions of relationship fulfillment at many and all levels. We are seeing *the necessity of complementation*—the Moon is necessary to reflect the light of the Sun—the essence of relationship, the outreach of idealized projection, and *the measurement context of reality.*

4

INTIMACY THERAPY

Getting Past the Fears

Many people live their life without understanding it. Jung's insight that we need others to know ourselves is poignantly on target. The Yang *needs* the Yin. The Eastern half of the horoscope *needs* the Western half.

I feel that we owe it to the creative principle that gives us life to appreciate what we are about, from whence we have come, what we bring with us, and where we are going into the future. Being so concerned with life after death should not be at the neglect of life after birth.

This does not mean we should pursue unrelenting scrutiny and overanalysis of all experience and thought, which can easily fragment and deaden life rather than invigorate and inspire it. Instead, it means seeing clearly the development of values, the growth of talent, the focus of motivation, and the reciprocal, cooperative relationship with others. Security within this understanding, within this development, builds the base for intimacy.

We all develop fears in our growing up process. These are *understandable* anxieties, part of the growth process, points of psychophysical caution. One emotional experience will link itself to other experiences. These experiences will become triggers for emotional response. This process repeats constantly. The experiences

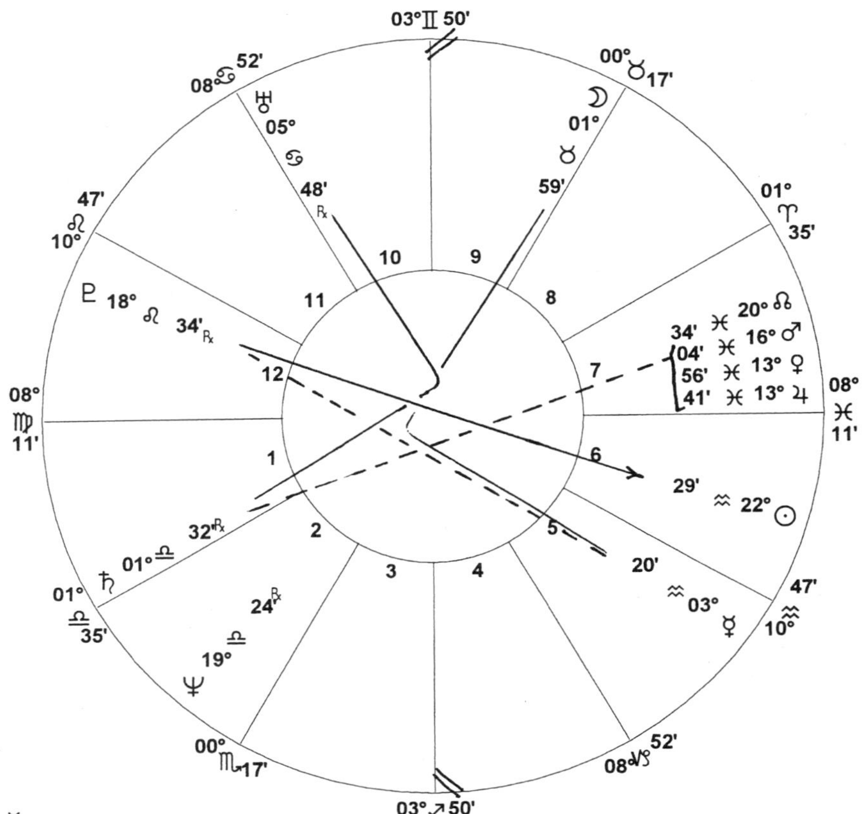

♇ = ♄/♅

	☽	☉	☿	♀	♂	♃	♄	♅	♆	♇	☊	Mc
☉												
☿	□a 01°22											
♀												
♂	∠s 00°54		∠s 02°16	☌a 02°09								
♃				☌s ∥ 00°14	☌s 02°23							
♄	⊼s 00°27		△s 01°49		q a 00°27							
♅	✶a 03°50	⚼s 01°40	⊼a 02°28				□s 04°16					
♆		△s 03°05			∥							
♇		☍s 03°55	q a 00°14		⊼a 02°30		∠s 02°02	∠a ∥ 02°14	✶s 00°50			
☊			∠a 02°13	☌a 06°38	☌a 04°29	☌a 06°52			⊼a 01°09	⊼a 02°00		
Mc			△s ⋕ 00°30				△s 02°19		⚼a 00°34		Qs 01°17	
Asc		q s 00°42		☍a ⋕ 05°45		☍a 05°30		✶s 02°23				□a 04°21

Chart 12

"David"

force us into behavioral routines—usually defensive—and enduring mindsets, the structure of which defines our personality.

How we learn to understand that process, become objective in appreciating it, and to rest realistically and confidently upon that knowledge in order to grow forward—that is the poise we need for intimacy and its rewards.

Chart 12: "David"

"David" is fifty in 2001. Here is an analytical outline of his horoscope (p. 84):

- The orientation is conspicuously to the West, "giving the self to others." This supports the Sun-Moon blend: "a closed-in involvement between the intellectual and the emotional. Personal development is the most important thing in life. The challenge is to find social application of all the special understanding one has."
- Pluto opposes the Sun: somehow, there is a "blanket over David's hand grenade," something that suppresses his special understanding, slows down his humanitarian orientation, his mission.
- There is the Saturn$_{Rx}$ phenomenon, at the Aries Point, squared by Uranus, and quindecile with Mars. Saturn rules the 5th and Mars rules the 8th, and we can expect some manifestation of the suppression within giving love and managing sex within relationships, the latter reflecting the former.
- The sensitivity is enormous (Mars-Venus-Jupiter triple conjunction in Pisces): Neptune, ruler of the 7th, is in fine shape: relationships should not be difficult, but *something* is suppressing the natural sensitivities, the social message: are the mind and the emotions fighting together? What might be within that struggle?
- Mercury, ruler of the Ascendant and the Midheaven, is quindecile with Pluto (in its key opposition with the Sun) and Mercury is semisquare with the Nodal Axis, *the closest aspect in the horoscope*: the mind is caught up with the "blanket" (the suppression) and it could

be linked to the mother, a companion observation along with the paternal reference of Saturn retrograde.

- The Mercury square with the Moon (besides promising articulate volubility) also begins to show the maternal influence as well.
- There is no Fire articulation in David's horoscope: here is a weakness in motivation, in drive, liveliness, thrust forward.
- Finally, a powerful Midpoint Picture adds a special dimension to the analytical orientation: Pluto=Saturn/Uranus, *"a tremendous fear of loss, a haunting fear."*

David's father was a strong, scary, "Shut up and do what I say" father. David's mother showed him in subtle ways that she really never wanted to be a mother. David said he could remember his hot-tempered mother often driving off temperamentally and his father saying that he had no idea where she was going, i.e., the implication was clear that perhaps she wouldn't come back and this introduced the primal archetypal fear of abandonment.

David spoke about his mother and father emotionally, often, pointing out how his father had been abandoned by *his* father, "He just went away and never came back." It was not difficult to hear the accumulating instances and feelings about abandonment; and the midpoint picture Pluto=Saturn/Uranus gained focus (tremendous fear of loss; upheaval to protect assets; rebellion).

I asked David if he had ever seen his parents affectionate to one another. He said that he had, but that "neither parent had ever shown him their vulnerability. I never heard either one of them say, for example, 'I feel sad.'"

It was clear to me through the quindecile between Saturn and the triple conjunction in Pisces in the 7th (the orb with Jupiter-Venus is dissolved by the conjunctions with Mars) that David's *anima projection* was suppressed somehow, modified, thwarted, disillusioned, imploded. This probably occurred through the modeling of behavior for him by his parents: "David, I think all this curtailed your expression of the gentle, the emotional." That projection, that hope, that need, had been thwarted, and remained unfulfilled.

This was a major deduction, and David took it to heart.

David knew much about this situation. He was extremely articulate and appeared on top of it: "I can assure you that resolving my mother issues has been a major accomplishment for me. Breakups with women would invariably trigger very deep sadness, almost desperation in me [the negative anima], that I knew were partly about my erratic mother and what I feel were my abandonment issues. . . . Two years after I went off to college [Tr Neptune opposed his Midheaven, tr Saturn conjunct his Midheaven], my mother suffered a serious depression, becoming very suicidal."

I asked David how he had learned so much about his situation, and he told me of having seen a therapist and studying his dreams with her. "My mother was coming up in my dreams really often! The therapist actually asked me if I was *married* to my mother!"

When David and his first wife divorced, much pain emerged within him; aloneness, weeping, so many anxieties flooding out through his newfound understanding. It was quite moving—and a quite recovered and healthy indication—when David said, "It was then that I learned my Life Lesson: to be compassionate *with myself*"—a major statement of the Water element (Mars-Venus-Jupiter conjunction in Water in the 7th House). This means, of course, to know himself better, his vulnerabilities, to see them as natural and residually whole-making as the confident self extends itself anew to relationship.

At the end of our discussion, I worked with David to organize several points: "What principles helped you 'resolve your mother issues,' David?" I asked. Here is our short, most instructive list:

1. David got the legacy of abandonment fears up and out, dredged them up within the time period of his divorce. Getting them up and out allowed him to manage the fears; *he saw what they were.*

2. In managing the feelings and thoughts, David gained conspicuous objectivity about the mother/father situation.

3. Learning the traffic pattern within those emotional reactions and the values involved with them gave David the poise to respect who he was.

4. And finally, David learned that he need not fear showing his sensitive, feeling self to someone else; he *could* talk openly about love; he did not need to see relationship within the fear-perspective of abandonment but within the complementation that could support further growth and fulfillment. He could get on with his mission to help others with his sensitivities and talents. David is becoming a fine astrologer.

The final part of our discussion dealt with the need for Fire shown in the horoscope, for a relationship that would provide those energies. This would help make him whole.

David said that he had had two relationships with Aries women, but they never worked out.

"Did you resent their leadership?"

"Yeah! I think you could say that!"

"The resentment might have been wanting to give your mother a second chance, if you will, not giving life over to their Aries leadership."

"Yeah. Interesting. Perhaps I had to go through that phase. Now I want someone who is closer to me temperamentally."

"Well, the lady with whom you are now in relationship, is it close?"

"Yes, very."

This lady has one Fire point of emphasis: Jupiter in Aries; here is the strong positive-thinking complement to David's need. The rest of her astrology is strong Water-Air.

"I would suggest, then, David, that this relationship is excellent for you because the leadership she contributes is ameliorated by the softer dimensions. It's easier to take."

David agreed.

Here is the case where David's anima projection through Venus in Pisces (emphasized in the triple conjunction) and the need for the Fire Element finally have met in the blend of his lady's astrology.

Chart 13: "Gwen"

"Gwen" is our next case (p. 90). She is fifty-five in 2001 and has been married three times (plural marriages can be anticipated when Gemini or Pisces is on the Descendant; this is an old-time rule that seems to hold up a lot of the time) and had "many relationship adventures." She is in yet another relationship at present and is very happy within it. Gwen says, "I feel I have been able to overcome a lot of my relationship problems, but maybe I have just worked out a comfortable compromise."

With regard to relationships, this horoscope is deceptive at first: Mercury, ruler of the 7th, is in Libra and is very nicely aspected with a quintile to the Moon and a trine to Uranus. But, when we begin to look further we discover Uranus is quindecile to the Ascendant, a tremendous anxiety about who one is, how the identity is forming and a search for self-confirmation through relationship [Uranus in the 7th]. A lot of emphasis is being placed on relationships.

Venus is peregrine in Scorpio, in the 12th. It is also at the Sun/Moon midpoint, a vital, potentially dominating position in every person's horoscope. This Venus is extremely strong, and extremely vulnerable to unfulfillment, being in the 12th and representing relationship judgment that will probably be swamped with emotional intensity. There is the potential here of conquest to prove the self. [Note that Venus (and the Sun/Moon midpoint) are in quincunx (adjustment pressure) with Uranus.]

We then see that Jupiter, ruler of the Ascendant, is conjoined with Mars and squared by Saturn. This indicates yet again some developmental difficulties. And all of this is taking place with a conspicuous Southern Hemisphere emphasis, promising easy victimization, being pushed around by circumstance.

The Sun-Moon blend promises a tie-in between the energy to please and gain appreciation (Libra) and the needs to make things happen, get things done (Capricorn). This is the blend of the "people manager." But all of this is idiosyncratically directed (Moon in the 1st) to proving who *Gwen* is. As well, Neptune is conjunct the Sun, and Neptune is Oriental (rising last before the Sun does): this promises a powerful life-driving idealism.

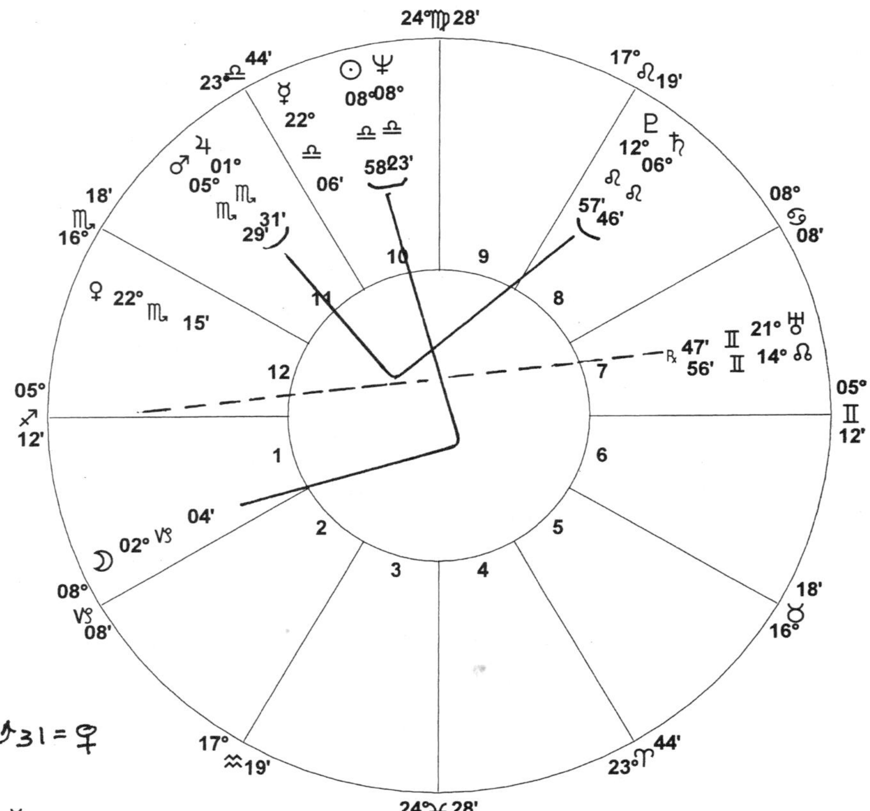

☽ 20♏31 = ♀

♀ = ☿/♅

	☽	☉	☿	♀	♂	♃	♄	♅	♆	♇	☊	Mc
☉	□a 06°54											
☿	Qa 02°02											
♀		∠s 01°43										
♂	✶a 03°26											
♃	✶s 00°33				☌s 03°58							
♄		✶s 02°11			□a 01°17	□a 05°15						
♅			△s 00°19	⚻s ∦ 00°27	⚼a 01°18		∠a 00°01					
♆	□a 06°19	☌s 00°35		∠a 01°08			✶a 01°37					
♇		✶a 03°59		∦			☌a 06°11	∥				
☊		△a 05°58		∦		⚼s 01°35		☌s ∥ 06°52		✶a ∥ 01°59		
Mc				✶s 02°14				□s 02°41	∦			
Asc		✶a 03°46	∠a 01°54				△a 01°34	q a 01°35	✶a 03°11			Qs 01°16

Chart 13

"Gwen"

About idealism, Gwen said that she had totally unrealistic (Neptune) expectations for men and relationships [an animus profiled in part by Sun conjunct Neptune]. She had taken her cue from movies, television, and novels. "I really thought the love of a good woman could overcome all odds [the negative male experience] and, once you were in love, everything would fall right into place."

Gwen also thought that she had to behave in an idealized fashion by always being nice, pretty, sweet, and obliging (the social norm for females). It has been only in the last eight years or so that Gwen began to accept men as real human beings and to quit expecting them "to be Clark Gable, Jimmy Stewart, or James Garner." She also learned how to deal with the inevitable conflicts in relationship, the bubbles bursting. In short, she learned *realism*.

Gwen's dominant Venus (peregrine, at the Sun/Moon midpoint at 20 Scorpio 31) rules her 11th House: Gwen was dominated by proving who she was (Uranus quindecile the Ascendant) in terms of being loveable (11th House). Everything had to fit an ideal. [Additionally, this thought is synthesized completely in the midpoint picture Venus=Mercury/Uranus, the tendency to love spontaneously, to gain self-confirmation over-exaggeratedly through relationship.]

How had these feelings and behaviors accumulated within Gwen's identity? The Neptune conjunction with the Sun in the 10th, Neptune ruling the 4th, highlights a parental influence for sure. The key Uranus in its tension with the Ascendant is square to the Midheaven. The Sun-Neptune conjunction is square the Moon, and brings *the mother to our attention*. [Normally, within this pattern there is a strong Nodal contact, bringing the mother into consideration dramatically, but the orb here of Node-Uranus is too wide to be sure.]

Gwen focused strongly with me on the issue of her not feeling loveable, and she focused strongly on her relationship with her mother. Gwen's mother never told her she was loved: "It was just the opposite, and I withdrew. When I was naughty, for example, she used to say to me, 'Who are you? You're not my little Gwen! Go away!'"

I suggested that perhaps the mother was jealous of Gwen's relationship with her father. Gwen said, "I was so close to my father; there was jealousy, I'm sure."

The feelings of being unloved/unlovable taken on through many behavioral interactions with the mother *were carried over into Gwen's relationships with others.* "With every man I was with, I doubted he loved me. I thought marriage would solve that problem, fitting the ideal, etc., but it didn't."

During our discussion, I asked Gwen about a key time in 1964, when she was just eighteen [SA Mars=Venus; SA Uranus=Sun-Neptune, exact at age seventeen]. Here was an enormous punctuation of all her love concerns: Gwen was at college and pregnant, had a miscarriage, and suffered guilt/shame for a long time thereafter. She had been "naughty," and this translated into being unlovable.

Now at age fifty-four, Gwen has settled down. She feels she is finally beyond those developmental problems—"or I have just worked out a comfortable compromise?" How did she do it?

I asked Gwen if she had ever been to a psychotherapist to get some help on all this [Pluto in the 8th so very, very often suggests such determined self-study]. She said that there had been a few visits, talking about her and one of her son's problems, but, in the main, she had a female friend with whom she could discuss anything under the sun! That friendship has lasted some thirty years and is still going strong.

"My friend has served as a *nonjudgmental, unconditionally loving confidante and counselor for me all these years, as I have been for her.* We were just saying last week that we didn't know where we would be today without each other. When someone you care about knows your deepest secrets, sees you at your absolute worst, accepts and loves you and *makes no value judgements*, phenomenal healing can take place." ***What an extraordinary description of intimacy and its rewards!***

One's best friends become "family," and these friends can be more powerfully significant than one's blood-ties.[33]

33 Sullivan, *Dynasty*, chapter 7, "Families and Our Familiars," 138.

Through her intimate friendship, Gwen (1) brought up and out the inner information and experience evaluation within her development. Then, (2) objectification was possible, she could see the mother situation and understand it from her perspective and from her mother's. (3) She gained poise to respect who she was, through her own eyes first and then through the regard of her friend; and finally, (4) to extend herself on realistic terms to others in her world . . . no more bubbles to burst.

What's Love Got to Do with It All?

Love is a story. It is developed by many authors, presented with many themes, but focused on one singular ending of happiness ever after. Wanting to find love, hold on to it, keep it strong and enduring is a tremendous burden to relationship.

The scenario of love begins soon after our birth. The first question the baby hears that imprints itself on the brain is "Do you love your mommy?" To reward the expectations of the parent(s), getting to say the word "love" as soon as possible is extremely important. Love ties us to the significant other, attracts rewards from someone else, and gives us the feeling that we are living correctly.

Then we witness—perpetually, unconsciously, consciously—the love modeling between our parents. Do they love each other? How do they show it? Does it delight or embarrass me? Why? How do I fit in? Do they still love me in spite of what's going on? Did they ever?

What happens, of course, is that "other things" take place in the family experience; the child is taken away from center stage. Another child might take its place there; parents become preoccupied with their work, their relationship suffers. Early socialization then exposes the child to what other children feel and think; there is competition among the children; values are established; the teacher becomes the first extension of the parent(s) outside the home. Does the child feel loved by others? Does school performance—the child's emerging image—interest the parents?

Television, movies, magazines, books come into the development of this thing called love: how important it is, how desirable it is; how people show it. Am I loveable? Perhaps I don't feel it anymore. My parents have forgotten about it. And now we're moving, and there's a new school, new friends; I've got to start all over again. No one really cares.

Astrologically, the self-worth concerns suggested by the condition of the 2nd House, especially through its ruling planet, are always in developmental square to the affairs of the 5th House, the giving of love. The 5th House derived from the 7th is others' giving love to us; therefore *the 11th is the experiential zone of love received,* hoped for, anticipated, assumed. The 8th House is the second of the 7th, the self-worth concerns of others in a face-off with our own concerns in the 2nd.

This Grand Cross of love concerns is crucial. Difficulties suggested here are easily transferred to the 7th through rulership networks, as we have seen often in our example cases. In playing out the love scenario, we must involve the 7th House, relationships. So very easily, we transfer to relationships the anxieties built up within our early home experiences: feelings of not being loveable are played out in relationships. Love often vanishes because it is not believed.

The 5th House of giving love is in supportive sextile to the 7th. But if there is difficulty with reference to the 5th the supportive relationship is hard to achieve. Relationships suffer. The developmental tensions back up through the networking and our self-worth insecurities are exacerbated, etc. Old anxieties play themselves out again; unfinished business in the early home reigns front and center in adult life.

What has happened? The idealistic love projection, seasoned by Hollywood, by thousands of popular songs, by dreams, driven by hormones, competitively paralleled with the love experiences of our friends, this projection upon the significant other, the chosen one, the perfect one—the animus/anima projections—is undermined. The bubble bursts. Reality exposes and represents failure. Love is lost.

So often in the love-at-all-costs scenario, we sacrifice to the quest our individual needs, the need constructs that define us individually. In the main, the man's needs usually prevail, according to societal construct; the female's needs are secondary, more compliant, and more patient in their press. Love is to make us whole, to complement one person with another, to make each more when together than when either is alone, to complete the horoscope. But, under enormous tensions to live the story, the individual tends to lose Self, and less is brought into the relationship. We are unfulfilled.

And in that unfulfillment, we begin to blame the other person for the unhappiness that always accompanies underachievement of personal needs, when we feel personally incomplete. We feel guilt, the pain of feeling that we have not done our best to help fulfill the other's needs.

Rewriting the Story

All of these tensions that we see constantly to one degree or another in our client horoscopes are somehow, for some reason necessary in our growth. They *are* the "refiner's fire." They *are* how we become who we are supposed to be. Difficulty eventually builds strength. Ideals—our projections of the perfect love—are certainly motivational, but it is realism that makes the ideals practical.

In our society, in our families, we are not taught about these things. Somehow we are supposed to learn how to traffic the incredible demands of love relationships, explore sexuality, and organize self-confidence and trust to create intimacy *instinctively*. The mistakes that we make eventually must refine our approaches, teach us lessons, and, in some scenarios, eventually bring us happiness. If we knew more about all this early on, the process of becoming would not be so painful.

In growing up, we learn to deal with many different conditions linked to behavioral prescriptions put upon us by the outer environment, beginning with our family. We seek the soul mate, the one who will love us and attract our love *unconditionally*, free from the fear of criticism, devaluation, of *not* being loved, of being rejected and abandoned.

It is fair to observe that two people meeting and exploring the potential of loving each other begin by looking into each other's eyes. They get lost from the world by searching one another for safety.

In a realistic view of love, perhaps it is better for two people to look together into the *same* direction, to follow the same path—away from the Hollywood passion ideal that is practically impossible to sustain. Then, the togetherness is complementary rather than consuming. Each individual is respected, and the pair gains strength; one person is the appreciating mirror for the other.

In our times now, the love story is being rewritten. Individualism is rampant in modern culture. "Doing your own thing" has gotten out of hand: since 1960, the divorce rate has doubled (now every other marriage ends in divorce), violent crime has quadrupled, and projections for depression this year are ten times what they were forty years ago. People appear more successful, more affluent than ever before, but they are unhappier, lonelier. Yet the primal drive to complete oneself through a love bond with another is inexorable; unions are pursued now more in desperation than in romance.

The answer is to learn about love wisely rather than passionately—and the sooner in life the better. Love must facilitate partnership. Respect of individualism between two people looking in the same direction will allow intimacy *when the mutual respect pushes criticism away*. Personal shortcomings are not ignored; rather, they become part of the realistically bound profiles. Discussion hides nothing, but everything that defines the individual is welcomed and respected.

In this process, complementation (led by astrological element need and gain) builds strength. Synastry shows togetherness and teamwork. Love is comfort rather than burden.

Moon-Marriage Orientation

With the whole thrust to love and make a connection, to relate in order to become whole, while still preserving the growth of ourselves as individuals, it is clear that we relate and we marry *to fulfill the reigning need of our personality.* Using the Sun's energy, we grow into and through life in terms of the Moon motivation to fulfill its psychodynamic complex. The compatibility between one person's resources accumulated in the fulfillment process and the other person's resources is what sparks interest between two people, inspires a try at intimacy, and can support love, looking together as a unit into the same direction for further growth.

The Moon in Capricorn will marry—all things considered, of course—for fulfillment of getting things done, a practical orientation within life, where progress *is* the most important product of the relationship.

The Moon in Aquarius will marry for something special, some unique sense of mission, often socially related, that would make the marriage different, exciting, even avant-garde. Uniqueness as a unit will probably be the key concept.

The Moon in Pisces will marry to be fulfilled within his or her sensitivities, appreciating the romance and ideals of understanding and sharing, perhaps on the inner plane as much as on the outer, certainly involving the intuition significantly.

The Moon in Aries will probably marry to be very important. The partner will have to offer ego reflection that is very strong, dramatic, and credible.

The Moon in Taurus will need to marry into a structured rightness, a way of protecting progress against change, hedging against transient insecurity.

The Moon in Gemini will need a cerebral base for a good marriage, a union in which diversity, thought, effervescent discussion, and a certain amount of indecision will be appreciated.

With the Moon in Cancer, the marriage potential will be based foremost on emotional security, the truth of love, especially in the home, within the sense of family. This will have to be clarified before trust can bloom.

With the Moon in Leo, the marriage will be one to serve the need to be the hero or heroine! The marriage must support the aggrandizement of self-importance and magnanimity.

The Moon in Virgo will marry to fulfill the need of being proper, correct, right. Mind will prevail over emotions.

The Moon in Libra will marry for social exposure, for relationships through the marriage out to other publics. A certain amount of aesthetics will be required as well.

The Moon in Scorpio will marry with the sense of control, perhaps even possession being very important. A deep privacy or secrecy will be a protected right even within an open bond.

The Moon in Sagittarius will marry for the personal opinions to be respected, for ego to be recognized for energy, learning, and diversification.

These Moon orientations combined with the condition of the 7th House ruler and any strong aspects to the Moon (etc.) delineate reliably the drive and operation of the marriage instinct.

In the horoscope, we must never forget that the horizon line with "relationships" to the West, in the 7th House, anchors itself at the Ascendant, the center of our individuality. When a major Arc or Transit relates to the seventh cusp, the Descendant, *it also relates to the Ascendant.*

When Neptune contacts the seventh cusp (or any Angle) there is high probability that the time period of one to one-and-one-half years will correspond to ego-wipeout, some enforced retreat of the Self to gather new information, new energies, new understandings for growth. It is ordinarily a very difficult time in life.

Such a situation occurring during marriage years will imbalance the relationship. The Neptune is *opposing the Ascendant*, the center of Self is being blanketed somehow, and the effect from this will be focused in the marriage (the seventh cusp). This imbalances the marriage; the bubble may burst; the ideal may be shattered; difficulties may emerge through previous unknowns about the spouse emerging dysfunctionally in marriage consciousness. If the spiritual or gentler dimensions of the marriage bond (with reference to the need complexes of the two individuals) are well developed, this Neptune time may be positively reinforcing. Ideals may be strengthened with good cause; aesthetics may bloom in the union; the sense of spiritual or religious discovery may reinforce the bond.

When Uranus contacts the seventh cusp, *the Ascendant will be intensified as well.* The individual will become more emphasized. Again, this may imbalance the routined positions and way of the marriage. One person may be outgrowing the other and the significance of the bond. This is why the planet Uranus figures so often in divorce or separation (or going into business for oneself; running away, escaping, etc.). The marriage must make space and place for this specially developing partner whose development pace is peaking.

With Pluto contact with the seventh cusp, opposing the Ascendant, we can expect a power struggle in the marriage. New perspectives may beckon and the decision-making process about following one or the other is out of balance. For the two persons to look together in the same direction, a new orientation is being commanded.

When Saturn contacts the seventh cusp, there will probably be a shift of gears in the marriage to accommodate the strategies of work and development. Has ambition gradually but definitely outdistanced mutual support?

With marriage, we seek to create a bond that will help us to fulfill our needs better than we can do alone. Part of our responsibility within the marriage bond is to recognize the individuality of the partner while looking together in the same direction for growth. Helping our partner grow as an individual strengthens the marriage bond greatly. This is the challenge to Selfhood *and* Selflessness simultaneously. Sometimes it is possible; sometimes it is not.

Intimacy is the precursor to deep relationship, or, in some cases, it is pursued in a loose relationship to make the relationship stronger. Intimacy is elusive because it requires *two* people to be well informed about themselves, honest about what they know about themselves, and eager to let each other be what he or she is. That's difficult.

Intimacy falls victim easily to . . . the great enemies of intimacy are . . . ***criticism, rejection, and the threat of abandonment***, or the intrusive efforts to change someone to fit expectations. For someone who is unsure of him or herself, the openness of intimacy is frightening: it is avoided, self-isolation follows, and relationship is denied.

Intimacy therapy requires self-understanding with objectivity and honesty. This self-understanding must go through the social filters of gender profiling, parental support or lack of it in early traffic problems in the home, and whatever is developed defensively and brought into early socialization experiences. This self-understanding helps a person be all he or she is, with a plan for further development. Part of this self-understanding is the recognition of personal needs and an appreciation that all other people are going through the same process in life.

The final step to achieve intimacy is willingness for partnership in realistic terms, so that there is no bubble—or fewer bubbles—to burst in relationship.

5

SEXUALITY

Dealing with Self-Confirmation

With this topic, it is important to define our terms, with their particular meanings related to our study here. "Sexuality" is any condition relating to sex; the adjective is "sexual." "Sex" defines the act of genital involvement between two people or alone with oneself. "Sexy" tells us about being attractive and alluring toward sex, appearing or behaving in a sexual way, or being personally aroused or arousing someone else.

One can be sexy but not sexual: provocative but nonresponsive.

Sex is *not* intimacy. Too often, especially among the young, sex is thought to be a confirmation of intimacy. Our language says euphemistically about the sex act, "we shared an intimacy" or "we were intimate together," but this is incorrect; this reference to intimacy is simply a diplomatic way of saying that two people had sex, that they engaged in a sexual act.

There are many problems with the sense that sex can *substitute* for intimacy, bringing people closer together. While rape is sexual, for example, it is not intimate. The nonorgasmic woman or the impotent male, as another example, finds special other values within sexuality that come closer to intimacy; through the confidence supported by love, especially among the older, they are protected from criticism, rejection, and the threat of abandonment.

Sexuality is part of the gender stipulations and expectations that issue from society concomitant with our birth, with our being named. How to respond to our hormonal drives is dictated by the culture along with how to be in love, and both prescriptions are idealized in many different ways, and they are decidedly problematic within reality. The word "romance" tends to cover everything here. Romance is very, very difficult since it requires intimacy, focuses upon love, involves sex, and defines the bonding of relationship.

We can refer again to the Succedent Grand Cross of Houses: the focus on the crucial development of self-worth, the 2nd House, involves predominantly the affairs of the 5th, 8th, and 11th Houses.

The 5th House is always trine to the Ascendant: it is the easy giving of oneself, the creative extension of who one is. It represents the children we create as facsimiles of ourselves. Psychodynamically, it is the concept of love given, of giving love in many, many different ways. It is the House of sexual resources.

I have long studied the allied hypothesis that the occurrence of sexuality in our lives issues mainly from the 8th House, because of the placement of Scorpio on that House in the natural distribution of signs. I cannot support that hypothesis. The 8th House issues from the 7th as its base orientation. It belongs to the concerns and resources of others. Indeed, the 8th House is important as the resources taken in from others thorough sex and other activities, at one level of interaction or another, but it is not *the* central focus of sexuality. The 5th House *is*, and the 8th House works together with it.

The 8th House is the self-worth second House of the 7th. It is the self-worth profile of others with whom we are in relationship. Psychodynamically, during interaction within relationships of any kind, the meeting of self-worth profiles is dynamic indeed: it determines the potential for resource exchange, for taking control or giving "it" away. It is the recognition of how valuable each of us is in relation to others, during sex as well, when two self-worth profiles are in special jeopardy.

The square between the 2nd and the 5th zones of experience alerts us to the fact that *our ease with giving love, sharing sexuality, participating in the sex act, is dependent upon our self-worth profile:* we must feel good about ourselves first before exposing ourselves nakedly to others. In other words, confidence is required before pursuing intimacy. Difficulties with self-worth can keep us from even accepting/believing a compliment. This shows how sensitive these issues are and how problems within them work against relating.

The assimilation of developmental tension among these Houses can range from a straightforward comfort with oneself and a keen sense of the evaluation of others to a weakened and fearful state of low confidence and a state of routinized self-protection by complex defense mechanisms. The Grand Trine, for example, establishes among certain behavioral faculties a closed circuit of protection that becomes a bastion of resistance against intimacy since it protects against the give and take of relationship.[34]

To fulfill our birthright, we must procreate. The process is complicated by societal structure designed to allay wanton conquest by the male and constant victimization of the woman (note the societal prescriptions of masculine and feminine roles). Keeping order requires varying degrees of suppression. Hormones don't react well to that. The mind faces bewilderment. The concomitants of our self-worth profile get confused. Relationships are strained. Because it is so intensely neurological and central to the act of self-confirmation, sexuality becomes a force to contend with that is very problematic. The resolution takes many, many forms.

It has been presented that when sexuality goes well in a relationship it is perhaps 5 percent of the relationship. When it goes badly, it becomes 95 percent of the focus of relationship concerns; it is symptomatic of problems elsewhere in the relationship, as we shall see in the final section of our study.

---

34 Please see "Defense Mechanisms," 643–645 and the Grand Trine, 234–302 in Tyl, *Synthesis & Counseling in Astrology.*

A generation ago, when we knew less about the human condition, the study of sexuality in astrology was repressed. It was barely recognized, and many problems within human development went without discussion, unobserved, and unresolved in client consultation. Now, our holistic understanding of development is considerably more informed and keen in conversational management. The sexuality profile must be studied in every horoscope; it is the arena in which many developmental problems and issues struggle for catharsis.

Chart 14: "Jane"

Chart 14 shows us the spreading and integration of problematic concerns throughout "Jane's" identity during development, with a central resolution focus in sexuality. At my request, after much discussion, Jane writes eloquently her organized view of her development, how the problems emerged, how understanding established perspective, and how self-worth dynamics improved throughout the process. Jane is herself now a superb astrologer, clearly strengthened by her own experience and gifted insight to help so many others help themselves.

Let's orientate ourselves quickly to Jane's horoscope:

- The conspicuous Eastern Orientation: defensive posture in life, internally or externally, or both. The question is "why is the defensive posture adopted within development?" This hemisphere emphasis is echoed by the Ascendant ruler, Venus, being under much developmental tension through the conjunction with Uranus. Venus and Uranus are the two rulers of the 8th and the 5th Houses, respectively: sexuality must be part of the discussion of anxiety and unique development.

- Pluto, ruler of the 2nd, squares Saturn, *ruler of the 4th*; obvious parental concern that must be discussed. This will directly introduce concerns about self-worth, since Pluto rules the 2nd and Saturn is placed there.

- Mars, ruler of the relationship 7th, is vulnerable in Pisces and is retrograde and opposes the Sun in the 12th House. Here is another

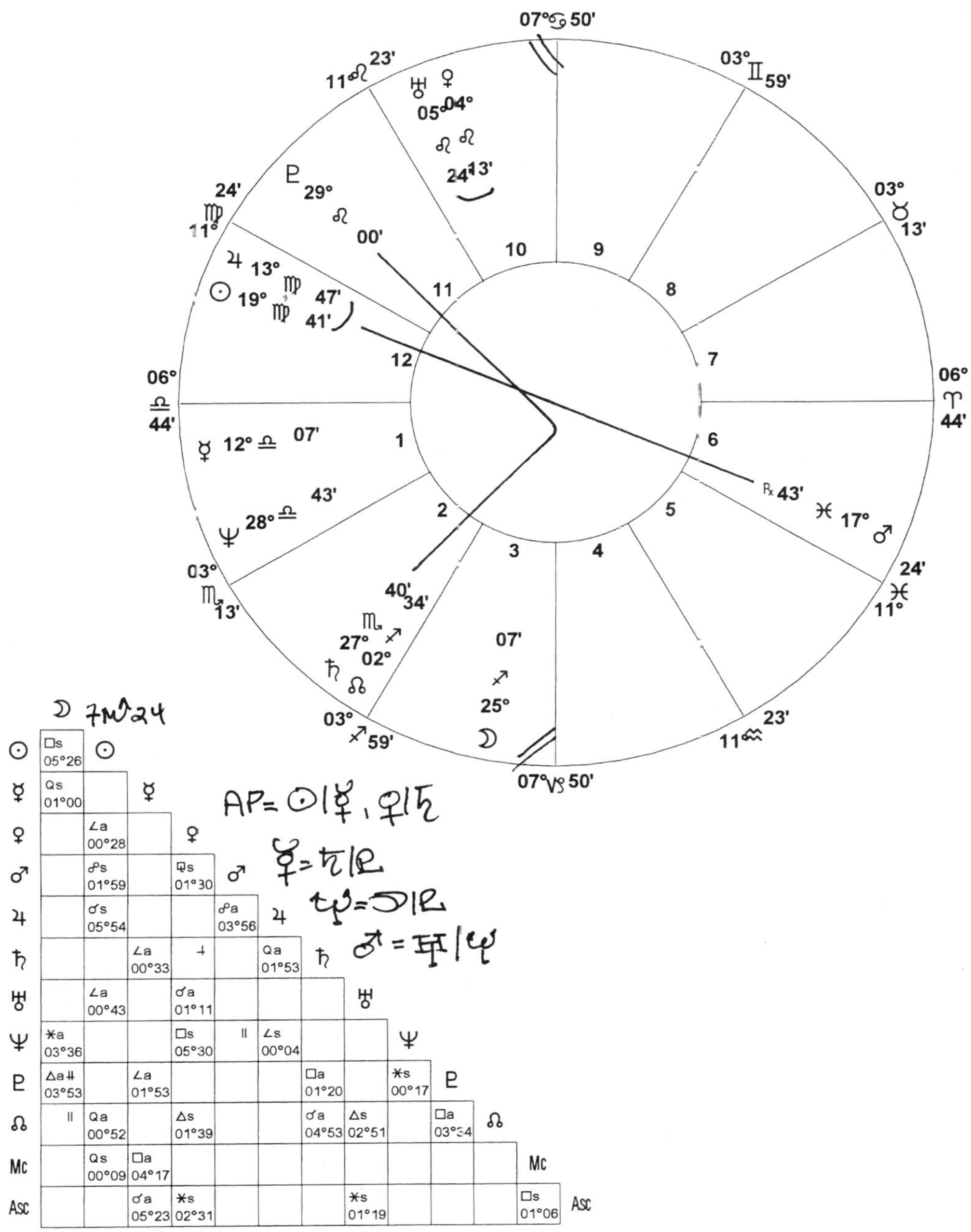

Chart 14

"Jane"

indication about relationship difficulty; the concept of retreat into defense is strongly suggested. As well, with the Sun ruling the 11th holding Pluto, a strong anxiety about being loveable is suggested.

- Mercury, ruling the 9th House of learning, of education, is peregrine and rising, giving it great strength. This observation is supported by Jupiter's rulership of the communication and mindset 3rd and its conjunction with the Sun, and the Sun-Moon blend: cerebral disposition to be correct and strong in the thrust of one's opinions.
- Several Midpoint pictures echo and reinforce general natal observations: AP=Sun/Mercury, Venus/Saturn suggest the cerebral, the communicative personality and the repressed emotional nature—both quite observable in social interaction. Mercury=Saturn/Pluto suggests depression. Neptune=Moon/Pluto, feeling weakened. Mars=Uranus/Neptune, applied creativity.

Jane writes her analysis as follows:

> Relationship and Intimacy Challenges—one of the biggest challenges I have faced in relationships has been overcoming a crippling sense of low self-worth and feeling ugly and unlovable. From a very young age (approximately seven), I was convinced that I was so ugly that "no one would ever marry me." [Note how Jane is phrasing this feeling at seven: in terms of fulfilling society's prescription that girls are pretty and girls get married.] No one ever disparaged my appearance, so I do not know how I came to believe this. I was *not* ugly, but truly believed that I was.
>
> My life has also been marked by abrupt and traumatic social and romantic rejections, starting from age eleven [tr Uranus and Pluto conjunct her Sun and tr Saturn conjunct her 7th] when a group of friends [Sun rules the 11th] I played with all "voted" not to let me play with them anymore, instantly making me an outcast [12th House feel]. This occurrence on the eve of adolescence confirmed for me that I was unattractive and would never be well liked. I went from being a fairly active and outgoing child to being withdrawn,

shy, and fearful in social situations. I had only one or two close girlfriends throughout high school, and never dated, never went to parties or dances. I was never socially a part of any peer group—not even the "nerds" or the "jocks"—of which I was both.

My emotional life was increasingly centered around romantic feelings for women. In high school I had intense crushes on women teachers and coaches. At age seventeen I became sexually and romantically involved with a girl my age, creating another social crisis in "belonging" and deepening my crisis of self-worth [tr Pluto conjunct her Ascendant]. I read some very negative material on homosexuality in my attempt to understand my identity and internalized the message that I was a very sick and disgusting individual. It took me years to recover from reading that. After two years, I dropped out of an Ivy League school because of my social distress [SA Mars=Asc, tr Pluto conjunct *Mercury*, ruler of the 9th].

I isolated myself within the gay subculture, hoping to avoid social rejection. Instead, I experienced divisive factioning and, once again, being outcast as undesirable from peer groups I belonged to. I looked to intimate relationships to bolster my sense of self-worth and give me a social connection I could not establish on my own. Yet, my self-worth crisis played itself out in relationships with alcoholics, physical abuse, verbal abuse, emotional and sexual distancing, chronic unfaithfulness, and some very painful rejections.

My fear of intimacy was a fear of rejection: *if you really get to know me, you will reject me.* I have suffered from deep feelings of shame about my appearance and my personality. Much of the healing I have experienced in these areas has come from relationships with lovers. I learned from one that I am physically attractive. I learned from another that I am a very special gifted person who has a lot to offer others. So, even as I have attracted some abuse and rejection into my life via relationships, I have also been blessed with love which has been deeply healing of my most painful wounds.

I have experienced a great deal of seemingly "irrational" rejection—sudden, traumatic breaks in relationships for no good reason.

> The most recent—a sudden, totally unexpected abandonment by my partner of eleven years [tr Neptune=Sun/Moon]—has been like a culminating lesson in living in a world of impermanence and changeability. In the aftermath of the break-up, I found myself living very much in the present moment.
>
> Guarding oneself against loss or abandonment does not prevent it—it only prevents one from experiencing the love which exists in the present. I began focusing on loving whoever I was with in the moment, as intensely as I could, whether at work, with a friend, on the bus, or in the grocery checkout line. So even though I often felt suicidal and devastated, this amazing love began to pour forth from me [Uranus rules the 5th and conjoins Venus; now free of the problems].
>
> Within a few months, the universe blessed me with a new lover—a person whose love reaches deep inside me and helps heal the wounds. I am finding myself giving and receiving love with so few defenses these days. When I get scared about what the future may hold, I ask myself, "Well, how are things *right now*?"
>
> If things are going well in the present moment, I am determined to just enjoy it. If the shoe is going to drop, I'll deal with it when it happens. Eventually it will; it's the nature of our mortal existence [Realistic, strengthening protection against the burst bubble]. In the meantime, I am going to love as if my life depended on it [Uranus, ruler of the 5th, conjunct Venus, ruler of the Ascendant]—love my partner, my clients, my family, my patients, my co-workers, and my friends. I am finding that in loving others [the balancing shift to the Western Hemisphere], I am beginning to *really* love being me and love living my life.

Jane has learned her life. Through objective, realistic, fair assessment, Jane has been freed through her self-study. Apparently, she does not fear criticism, rejection, and abandonment any more; she can manage it all; she can join in intimacy for fulfilling relationship at many levels of her busy life.

Chart 15: "Ken"

Chart 15 belongs to a young man of twenty-nine, "Ken," who works as a computer database administrator (Jupiter in Virgo conjunct Uranus, in the 3rd, quincunx the Midheaven, the only aspects with the Midheaven; Moon in Gemini opposed Mars in Sagittarius, ruler of the 10th). The horoscope has a distinct Eastern (defensive) orientation. The reason could very well lie with parental interaction since Mars and Venus (the parental rulers) oppose each other, and Saturn in the 10th squares the Ascendant.

The most telling dimension of the horoscope is the peregrine Sun, *ruling the Ascendant and the 2nd House of self-worth*, making no Ptolemaic aspect. This suggests a dissociated identity complex, one that is searching all the time for some meaningful tie-in with life around him. In this case, with the Sun in Cancer, the tie-in would surely be with development toward emotional home security. En route, there is decided tension about relationships since Uranus, ruler of the 7th is squaring Mercury, the mind, the nervous system, etc.

Finally, in the initial orientation, we see Pluto conjunct the Nodal axis, suggesting a struggle with the mother.

Ken said his father was a "manager," that he had no feeling and treated him like a hired hand around the farm. On one occasion with tr Saturn conjunct the Ascendant, the father practically beat Ken (aged seven) "to death."

Ken's relationship with his mother was "rough; there were no emotions; she was a reclusive alcoholic."

Ken was always, always alone. He developed asthma (Moon-Venus in Gemini opposed by Mars) and a nervous stomach (Mercury in Cancer squared by Uranus). When I mentioned the difficulties developing intimacy anywhere in any relationship, Ken laughed and said, "I have never been in a substantial relationship. I'm self-destructive. I get nervous about it (relating)."

Of course, as with Jane, these deep self-worth problems (peregrine Sun ruling the 2nd, Mercury under tension ruling the 11th etc.) will manifest strongly in the sexual profile. This anticipation is reinforced by the rulers of the 5th and 8th, Jupiter and Uranus respectively, being conjoined. From very early

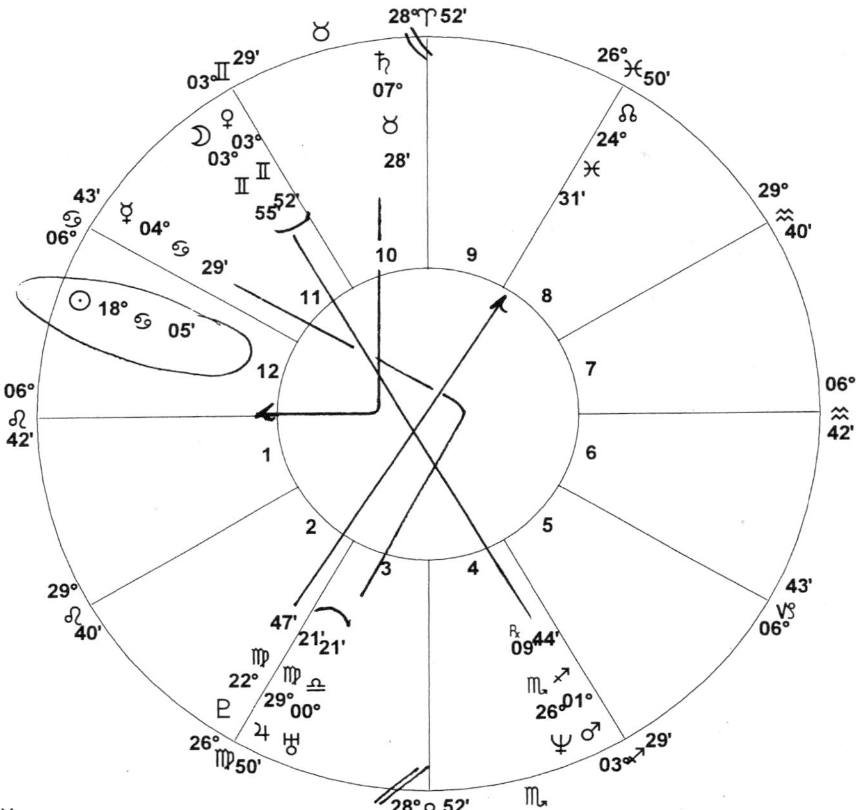

	☽	☉	☿	♀	♂	♃	♄	♅	♆	♇	☊	Mc
☉	∠s 00°50											
☿												
♀	☌s 00°03	∠s 00°46										
♂	☍s 02°11	⚼s 01°21	ǂ	☍s 02°08								
♃	△s 04°35	Qs 00°45	□s 05°08	△s 04°31	⚹a 02°24							
♄		Qa 01°23	⚹a 02°59									
♅	△s 03°34	Qa 00°16	□s 04°08	△s 03°31	⚹s 01°23	☌a ∥ 01°01						
♆				ǂ	☌s 05°36	⚹s 03°12						
♇						☌s 06°34	⚼a 00°19		⚹a ǂ 03°22			
☊						☍s ǂ 04°49	∠a 02°03	☍s 05°50	△s 01°37	☍a 01°44		
Mc						⚻a 00°29	∥	⚻a 01°30				
Asc	⚹s 02°47			⚹s ∥ 02°50	△s 04°57		□a 00°47			∠a 01°05		

Chart 15

"Ken"

on, Ken realized he was homosexual, but has necessarily been confined to a sex life of masturbation (often suggested by Moon-Venus aspects within a self-worth anxiety matrix; self-absorbed, self-confirming).

Ken lived long in loneliness, with no parental relational modeling whatsoever. He had no reference for his identity development. He said that when he entered the Air Force at eighteen (Sun=Ascendant; education interrupted, natal Mars conjunct Neptune ruling the 9th) he didn't think another gay person existed in the world!

Again we see the parental situation and the vulnerabilities to self-worth vagueness (2nd House), lovability anxiety (11th House), relationship difficulty (7th House) acted out in a difficult sexual profile. Ken will have to overcome the fear-of-criticism syndrome learned from his father's exploitation in order for intimacy to form and offer a possibility for meaningful relationship. Perhaps that is why Ken is looking for a father surrogate socio-sexually.

Chart 16: "Robin"

As a young man of thirty (Chart 16), "Robin" is a high-level accountant [the Virgo stellium; Mercury as final dispositor ruling the Ascendant and Midheaven, squaring the Midheaven].

There is a decided defensive orientation to the East surely linked to the father figure in the early home (Saturn retrograde quindecile Jupiter, ruler of the 4th). Robin's father was an alcoholic, often away from home, and, when there, tyrannical and wiped out. This "father" was Robin's adoptive father [note that Pluto was tightly conjunct the Ascendant, very often suggesting a birth anomaly; here, Robin was given up for adoption immediately at birth.]

Venus, ruler of the self-worth 2nd, is opposed by Saturn. This suggests the deep self-worth struggle in Robin's development. When he was very young, his adoptive parents were divorced. The adoptive mother remarried, and then this stepfather died of cancer.

Clearly we have many father issues unresolved. There is a clear father abandonment syndrome, and Robin—most intelligent and bright—knows it.

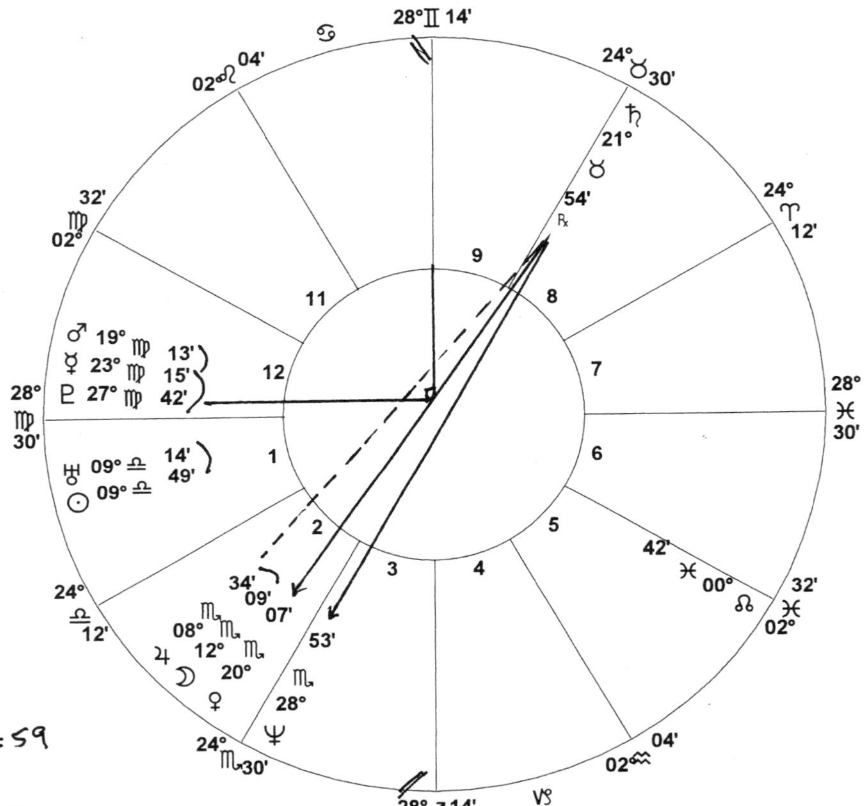

☽ 25♎59

M=♇|A
☽=♇|M
AP=☉|♂

	☽	☉	☿	♀	♂	♃	♄	♅	♆	♇	☊	Mc
☉												
☿		‖										
♀			⚹s 03°08									
♂			☌s 04°03	⚹a 00°55								
♃	☌s 03°36		∠a 00°18									
♄			△s 01°22	☍a 01°46	△a 02°41	q s 01°40						
♅		☌s ‖ 00°35					⚼s 02°20					
♆					Qs 02°19		☍s 07°00					
♇	∠a 00°33		☌a 04°27				△s ‖ 05°48		⚹a 01°11			
☊									□a 01°48			
Mc	⚼s 01°05		□s 04°59	‖					⚻a 00°39	□s 00°32	△a 02°27	
Asc	∠s 01°20		☌s 05°14						⚹a 00°24	☌s 00°48	⚻a 02°12	□a 00°15

Chart 16

"Robin"

Robin's understanding of these difficulties helped him "come out" as a homosexual at work and in his social life; he had been forced to understand and appreciate himself. Uranus rules the 5th and is oriental, rising last before the Sun, suggesting an independent, adventurous, confident, avant-garde spirit. In reference to his sexual profile within these family considerations, we could easily expect something different than the norm.

Robin spoke too much about two things: first, that his life was so remarkably improved now that he had "come out" at work and in his social life; self-aggrandizement. In other words, he was sure of himself—probably because of his excellent job performance and advance (MC=Pluto/Asc, Moon=Pluto/MC, AP=Sun/Mars)—and, second, that *he had found his soul-mate*, a gentleman with whom he knew he would be "for the rest of his life."

Robin was approaching his first Saturn return; he was facing a major high-level job change that probably would demand relocation (Saturn co-rules the 4th). So much in his reality was suggesting that the relationship would *not* prevail (with natal Neptune, ruling the 7th, squared by Saturn, as well). But the idealism was strong. It was clear that a great shock would soon be dealt to his self-objectification; it would build more maturity, and *then* perhaps, develop intimacy and love within a spiritually more fortified relationship choice.

The emergence of sexuality in the young life is an enormous burden: it presents a challenge to grow into adulthood, to confirm one's gender role and potential, and to begin to search for a partner, through love, expediency, or outright strategy. There are fears of breaking religious codes—even down to thinking about sex!, of being "caught," of disease, of impregnation, of failing.

All of this is opposed by new feelings of pleasure, the sense of confirming the self and its potential through masturbation, which in itself invites the development and repetition of special private erotic fantasies. These fantasies are as much discharge of tensions as orgasm is. We live another day for another buildup, another increment of age toward the time when everything will be legal, safe, expected, and free.

New problems present themselves: at eighteen, there is the big decision to go on to college or to go into the workplace, *or* to marry away from the household into one's *own* household and hoped-for freedom. If the education is interrupted [most usually in the American culture when the significator of the 9th House is under high developmental tension; triggered by an Arc or Transit complex at age eighteen to twenty] there is the suggestion that there was no parental preparation or push for going to college built into the young person's development plan. Is this also equated with the lack of parental caring, or just their lack of funds?

The precipitous marriage by male or female is a deeply disruptive occurrence within the American culture where a college education is the *sine qua non* of social and job mobility. The "train misses the station," so to speak. When will it circle around and get back on the right track?

Sexuality is often the drive here for precipitous marriage, justifying supposed early love. Sexuality is a powerful confirmation of self. Men seek to be proud of their sexual power; women of their sensual allure. The public media of our society fan the flames. In our society, there is no teaching or preparation for any of this. As the saying goes, we are left to our own devices.

In the exploration of early relationship, really early sexuality—and studies show how alarmingly early the explorations have become of late—values get confused. Without the maturity for intimacy, the young substitute sex for spiritual closeness, for understanding. The jolts of short-lived relationships jar the identity; they upset self-worth and lovability profiles. Defenses arise.

Chart 17: "Helena"

Chart 17, "Helena," shows yet again the defensive Eastern orientation combined with a Southern organization (above the horizon) suggesting the vulnerability to being pushed around, victimized, swept away by events outside her control.

Saturn exactly on the Ascendant is certainly severe, square the Moon (ruler of the 8th, part of the sexuality profile) and conjunct Mercury ruler of the

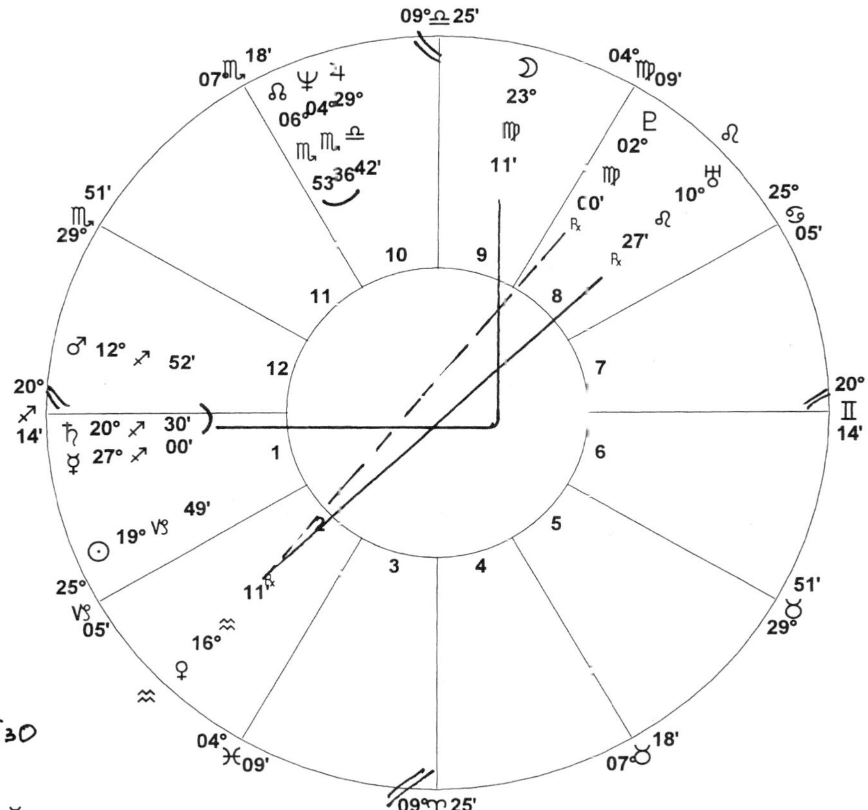

	☽ 21♍30	☉	☿	♀	♂	♃	♄	♅	♆	♇	☊	Mc
☉	△s 03°22											
☿	□a 03°49	∥										
♀												
♂		∥		⚹a 03°18								
♃			⚹a 02°42		∠a 01°50							
♄	□s 02°41	∥	☌s ∥ 06°30		∥							
♅	∠a 02°16		⚼s 01°33	☍a 05°44	△s 02°25							
♆						☌a 04°54	∠s 00°54	□a 05°51				
♇		∦	△a ∦ 05°00	q s 00°49	∦	⚹a 02°18	∦		⚹s 02°36			
☊	∠s 01°18	Qs 00°56		∥			∠a 01°23	□s 03°34	☌a 02°17			
Mc					⚹a 03°27		Qs 00°55	⚹a 01°02				
Asc	□a 02°57		☌a 06°46		∥		☌a 00°16		∠s 00°38		∠a 01°39	Qs 01°11

Chart 17

"Helena"

7th of relationships (difficulty here) and the 9th (high probability that education was interrupted).

Yet, Mars in Sagittarius usually suggests high opinionation needs, which without the credentialization of education lose audience and credibility. Mars in the 12th like this, usually within 10 degrees of the Ascendant, suggests strongly a complex of hidden anger. So we feel Helena swept away from herself somehow, nursing much anger about it, adopting severe, even depressing defenses, perhaps seeking out psychotherapy for help (Pluto in the 8th correlating very highly with seeking help from self-study, usually through therapy). *What has caused this?*

Saturn rules the 2nd House of self-worth. Mercury rules the 7th. This is serious.

Neptune, ruler of the mindset 3rd House, is conjoined with the nodal axis: here is the suggestion of the mother that must be pursued. This is echoed strongly by the Moon's square with Saturn and the Ascendant.

Venus rules the 5th and the parental Midheaven and is opposed by Uranus: there is much tension here. And *Venus is retrograde*, a strong statement of sexual concerns, a second agenda. Even further, Venus is quindecile Pluto, ruler of the love-received 11th. This suggests quite a complicated focus on the self-worth, giving and receiving love, sexuality areas. They could become obsessive.

I presented this to Helena gradually, gained corroboration every step of the way, and gradually Helena filled in the picture of her development reality.

Helena's mother had jumped off a bridge and committed suicide when Helena was fourteen. Helena's mother's mother had committed suicide as well, at the same age. Helena thought she had inherited a "suicide gene" and had done everything in her power thereafter, for the next twenty-nine years, to pattern her life differently than her mother's to avoid circumstances that could lead to her suicide as well! Here was the victimization by events, the self-demeaning agenda in her growth into womanhood.

She had gone into therapy at fourteen to try to work things out.

For the last seven years, Helena—who had never married and was now forty-three—had been celibate. I asked her why she had adopted this lifestyle, and she explained that she had been blessed with imposing good looks, superb figure, etc., and had grown weary of all the approaches she received from men; how she feared being hurt by them (perhaps part of her theorization about her mother(s) and their motivations for suicide; *and* she felt she had never been prepared for how to handle relationships. She said, "I've never had any formal training in that"—a perfect statement for a Capricorn with Saturn conjunct Mercury and the Ascendant in Sagittarius.

Recently, Helena had gone back to school—she had not gone to college before, since at that time in her life her father had remarried (at seventeen, tr Pluto conjunct the Midheaven with SA Pluto=(square) Asc-Saturn) and she had had a difficult relationship involving an abortion (at twenty-one, tr Pluto square Sun). In May 2000, she had just graduated with SP Moon conjunct her fourth cusp and SA Uranus=Moon in the 9th. She was on her way now to find her life.

Again, we see complications within the sexuality profile emerging from self-worth, giving and receiving love, and relationship vulnerabilities.

Intensity of the Sex Drive

The intensity of an individual's sex drive is conditioned by many variables, including hormone levels, the mind, nervous system engagement, socio-religious prescriptions, family modeling, self-image development, rewards and punishment, relationship history, idealization, fantasy, and more. For astrological analysis, it is helpful to ascertain the level of the sex drive *en route to discussion of possible manifestations there of developmental problems.*

Chart 18: "Laura"

"Laura's" horoscope (p. 118), suggests low-functioning sexuality. Here is how we see that: the 5th House is ruled by Venus, Venus in Virgo, and *Venus is retrograde*, suggesting some counterpoint, some other agenda regarding 5th

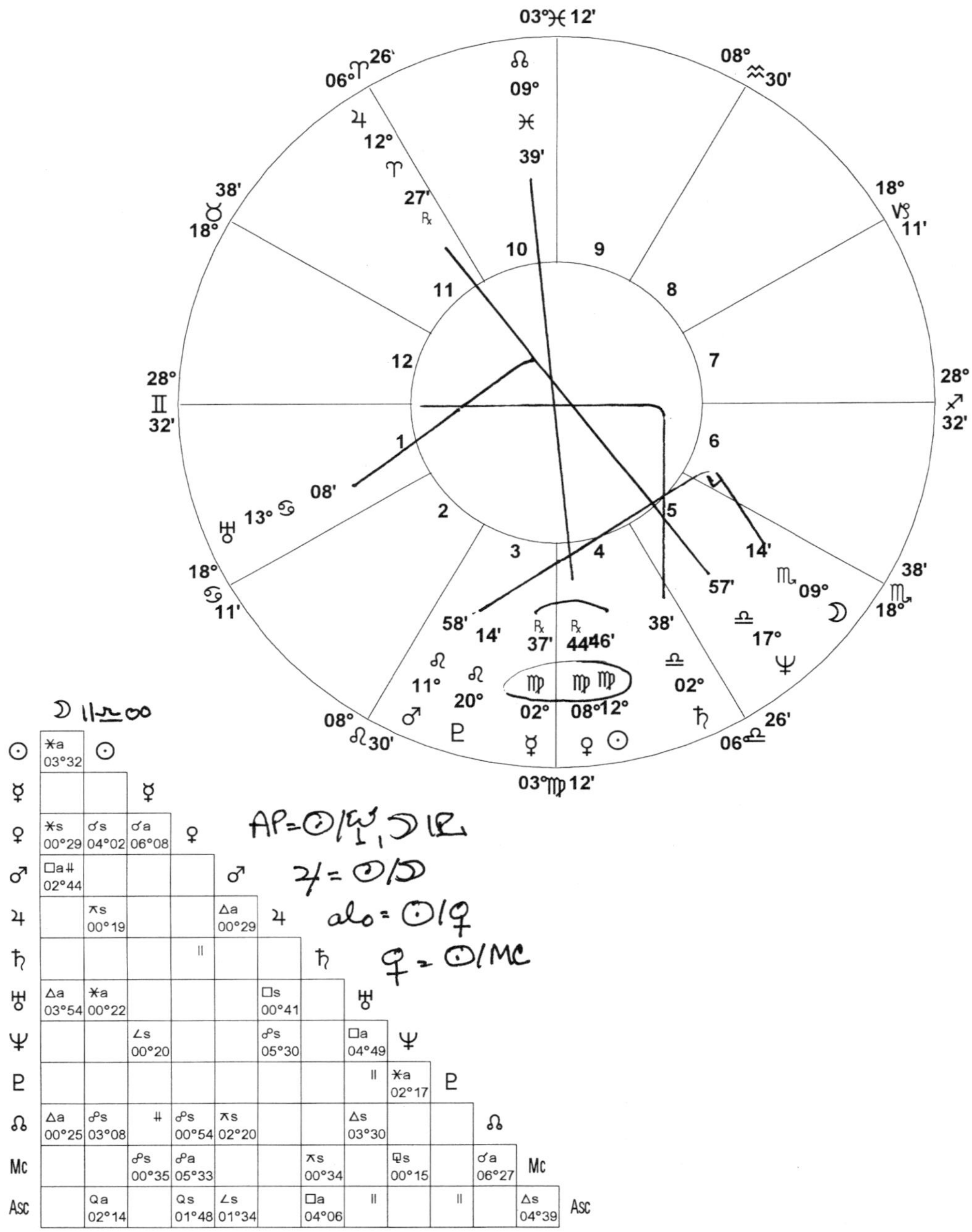

Chart 18

"Laura"

House matters. Venus is in the 4th, alerting us to one of the parents; it also rules the 12th, and there is a suggestion of limitations in the Venus need/behavior complex.

Saturn rules the 8th House and is peregrine, disassociated from the rest of the horoscope. Saturn is in Libra, disposited by Venus. This relates Saturn and Venus, and it is clear that there is something repressing sexual functioning, having children, an awkwardness with giving love.

Several midpoint pictures suggest an idealistic emphasis of values, echoing the natal Mercury-Venus, Venus-Sun conjunctions: AP=Sun/Neptune, Moon/Pluto (emotional zeal to outer targets); Jupiter=Sun/Moon (the dominance of learning and perhaps religiousness in development), Node=Sun/Venus and Venus=Sun/MC, a kind of "cozy" persona.

But what in the development fell into these sensitive areas—vulnerabilities—of the horoscope? Note that the Hemisphere emphasis is to the North, below the horizon, suggesting unfinished business in the early home; the Jupiter in Aries (a conspicuous ego orientation within reward needs) ruling the 7th is retrograde, opposed by Neptune, and squared by Uranus; and, finally, the high-focus Venus retrograde *in Virgo conjoins the Nodal Axis.*

"My mother was detached, distant, not available." Did she hold back from her husband? "Yes, she did." And that was your model? "Yes." And you do that too (hold back)? "Yes. But I've really been working on it. But, yes, for the first ten years of my marriage; yes."

Laura explained further: "In my childhood home, everything was a secret. There was little or no conversation and there was never a discussion. This, of course, spilled over into any kind of information exchange involving sex. If the subject came up, my mother would leave the room and the conversation would end.

"If she was mad at my father, she would go into her room, close the door and cry, while he stood outside the door looking helpless.

"It was very bizarre. I was always afraid, always defensive. There was no guidance; I hadn't a clue as to how to function in the world and relationships were disastrous . . . I hated myself [Note: Mars square Moon (mother symbol also), the ruler of her self-worth 2nd].

"Eventually I chose a husband who demanded that 'I play fair' . . . no passive/aggressive stuff. I loved him enough to work on myself and have grown enormously because of his influence. Now I have a lot of friends, I don't hate myself, and I have a marriage that has lasted twenty-six years."

Please look again at Helena's horoscope (p. 115), another case of low-functioning sexuality (seven years celibacy). As we have seen: Venus rules the 5th and is *retrograde*; the Moon rules the 8th and is squared by Saturn! The self-protecting device of celibacy was definitely tied up with Helena's extraordinary "suicide gene" complex. The mind set was completely caught up with this (Neptune rules the 3rd and conjoins the Nodal axis; the Moon is in cerebral Virgo [feelings into mind] and tied directly into the Ascendant by the square that includes Saturn and Mercury)!

Chart 19: "Violet"

"Violet" shows a high-sexuality need profile: Venus is in Scorpio (always a strengthened sexuality emphasis), rules the 5th, is squared by Mars and Pluto, *and is quindecile the Ascendant*, adding a dimension of compulsion, even obsession to the delineation. Sex defines who Violet is.

Saturn rules the 8th and opposes the sensitive, highly elevated Moon, ruler of her self-worth 2nd. Here is the key: a threatened self-worth profile strategically stimulating an overcompensatory sexual thrust for personal aggrandizement. Note the Gemini Ascendant, introducing the nervous system, the sense of variety, diversity, with Mercury, its ruler, *squared by Uranus*. This tells us that her nervous system is extremely involved with this complex; it relies on sexuality for reinforcement and composure [note the second agenda through retrogradation].

This Venus is supported well through the sextile with Jupiter, ruler of the relationship 7th. The $Mars_{11}$ square to Venus brings lovability into the

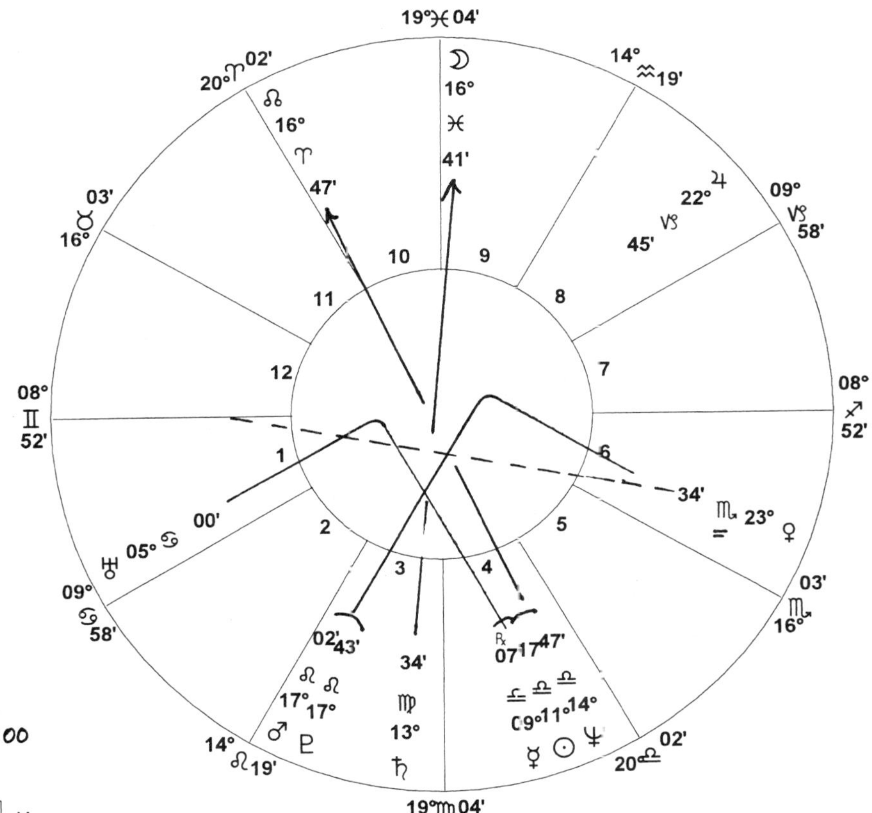

☽ 29♐00

		☉	☿	♀	♂	♃	♄	♅	♆	♇	☊	Mc
☉												
☿		☌s ǁ 02°10										
♀			∠a 00°33									
♂	⊼a 00°20			□								
♃				✶s 00°49								
♄	☍s ǂ 03°08			Qa 01°59								
♅		□s 06°17	□a 04°07									
♆	⊼s 01°55	☌a ǁ 03°30	☌s ǁ 05°40		✶s 02°15							
♇	⊼a 01°02			□s 05°51	☌a 00°41	ǂ		∠a ǁ 02°17	✶a 02°56			
☊		☍a 05°30			△s 00°15	□s 05°58			☍a 02°00	△s 00°56		
Mc	☌s 02°22	ǁ		△a 04°31	⊼s 02°02	✶a 03°41	☍s 05°30		ǁ	⊼s 01°21		
Asc		△a 02°25	△a 00°15	q s 00°17		⚻s ǂ 01°06	□a 04°42		△a 05°55			

♀ = ☉|♅

AP= ☉|☽, ♄ lolo, ☉|M,
☽|♅, ♃/A, ☽ lolo

Chart 19

"Violet"

portrait, driving the activity even further into pressing importance. The Pluto square to Venus is an extremely strong point of emphasis, leading easily to a conspicuous waste of emotions in the press to fulfill the deepest sensitivities (Moon in Pisces quincunx Pluto). And finally, Venus=Sun/Uranus, "out-and-out sexiness."

Note as well that we have a long string of Aries Point configurations. This tells us how "up front" Violet is with her being, with her need for sex to reinforce her ego constantly.

Violet is a very sensitive lady fighting a life-long battle royal with her mother, which battle is projected onto any other woman in her presence when a man is present too (the dramatic Saturn opposition with the Moon; the Nodal contact with Neptune then taken into the Sun and Mercury through the triple conjunction in the parental 4th).

Violet hates her mother. She professed throughout her life that she was really the daughter *of her mother's (other older) daughter (!),* impregnated by her father, with whom Violet had an intense relationship. It is valid here to suggest that Violet was doing away with her mother so that she could have her father to herself. The family had thirteen children in it, and Violet desperately needed to have her lovableness confirmed; her target was her father, her enemy was her mother. Later, in extension, Violet detested the mothers of her husbands.

When Violet married the first time, she had two children quite soon, and it appears she discovered her sexuality most intensely. Here was *the* way she could stand out from and away from other women. The obsession took hold.

At a family gathering with the thirteen siblings involved, all witnesses to this, Violet openly began to question her parents about their sex life. This was dramatic and shocking within this advantaged, solid family. It is almost as if she were asking for help, for the talkings-to she should have had long before. She was avoided, but the incident is still talked about almost thirty years later!

Violet, her husband, and her children moved away to a private school town, where her husband was a teacher. Violet says that she became "disappointed with her husband's penis" and she began having sex daily with students at the school. Her husband eventually sent her for psychological treatment, a scandal erupted, and the family was forced to move.

On vacations to visit members of her family, Violet would have sex continuously with many different men. She bought sex aids to use privately. Finally, the marriage ended in divorce.

Several affairs followed—but all the while, as a lawyer, Violet had constant employment, prestigious jobs, and, as well, constant sex with employees in every job situation . . . "hundreds." She was forced to leave several of these job positions.

Her second husband insisted on anal sex all the time: he did not want to have any more children since Violet detested his daughter from a previous marriage.[35]

She married again . . . to a younger workman in her older boyfriend's employ. She says quite openly that the attractive thing about this young man was his penis.

That marriage finally ended, and now Violet, at age forty-two, no longer practicing law, still obsessed with looking young, thin, and sexy, is in a sexless relationship with a much older man. The symbolisms throughout this drama of a charming, intelligent, highly sexual woman using sexuality obsessively for self-worth confirmation are so very clear; and so are her problems, the repeated search for and retreat to a father surrogate.

Chart 20: "Alfred"

"Alfred" shows a very strong sexuality profile (p. 124): note that Jupiter, ruler of the 5th is trine Neptune, ruler of the 8th. We can deduce that sexual expression will probably be working on a second agenda, since Mercury retrograde, ruler of the 2nd and 11th—two arms of the Succedent Grand Cross—is in the 8th and highly charged by the opposition with Uranus. The nervous system is highly involved here within the sexuality profile.

---

35 Clearly, this reasoning is a camouflage of some other motive since contraception could have been achieved differently.

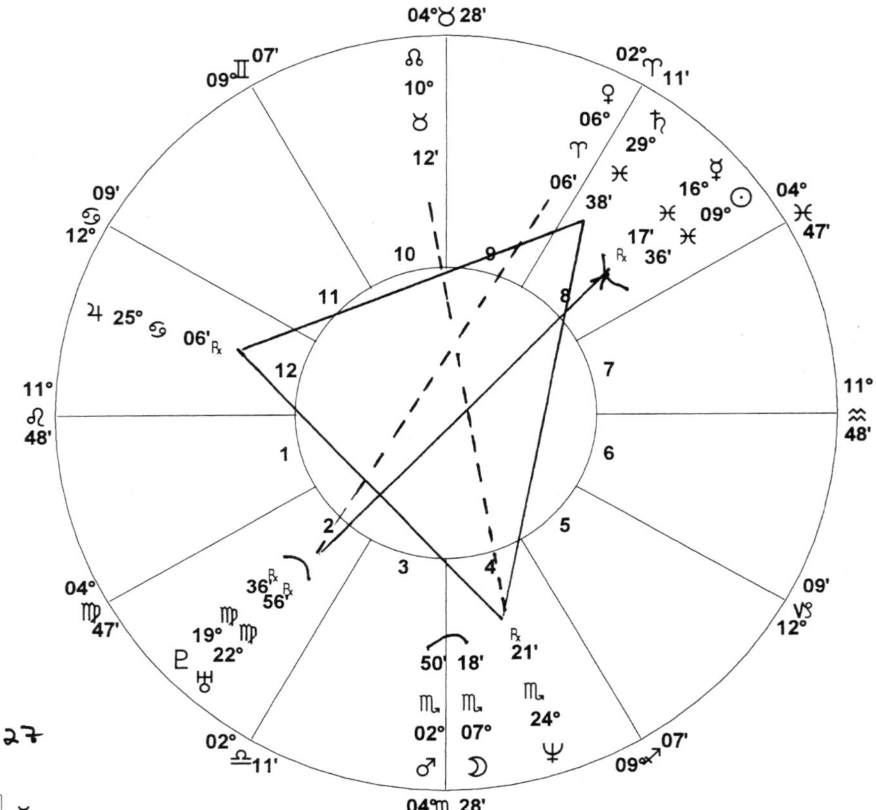

☽ 8♑27

	☽	☉	☿	♀	♂	♃	♄	♅	♆	♇	☊	Mc
☉	△a 02°17											
☿		☌a 06°42										
♀	⊼s 01°12		#									
♂	☌s 04°29		⚼s 01°32									
♃		⚼a 00°31										
♄			ǁ	☌s # 06°28		△s 04°32						
♅	∠a 00°38	q s 01°39	☍s 06°39	q a 01°50		⚹a 02°10	☍s 06°42					
♆						△a 00°45	△s 05°17	⚹s 01°25				
♇			☍s 03°18	q s 01°31	∠a 01°46			☌a 03°21				
☊	☍a 02°54	⚹a 00°37						⚼a 02°16	q a 00°51			
Mc	☍a # 02°50				☍s 01°38					⚼a 00°08	☌a 05°44	
Asc	□s 04°30	⊼s 02°13		△s 05°42					#	ǁ	□s 01°36	

Chart 20

"Alfred"

The picture of all this increases when we see Mars conjunct the Moon in Scorpio, and when we see Venus in Aries, *quindecile Uranus.* And, as well, the Water Grand Trine operating without the Sun or Moon (a closed circuit of emotional self-sufficiency, operating separately from the Sun Moon blend).

Masturbation is very important in his emotionally isolated life, his chief sexual outlet twice a day.

Chart 21: "Claudia"

"Claudia" (p. 126), also shows a highly active sexuality profile—certainly an area that would have to be discussed in consultation.

Note the stellium in Scorpio, with Mars conjunct the Sun, squared by Saturn, ruler of the self-worth 2nd. Here is a deep vulnerability that needs building up and confirmation—a process which so very often is sought through sexual activity. This is particularly urgent because of the Moon in Aries, the reigning need to be *numero uno.*

The Moon in Aries here rules the 8th House *and is peregrine*, and Venus, ruler of the 5th, is conjoined by Neptune. Experience supports that this configuration strongly suggests bisexuality or homosexuality.

The Scorpio complex and the Venus-Neptune conjunction relate to Jupiter, each by a quindecile, a compulsive or highly emphasized need press. Jupiter is ruler of the Ascendant.

Claudia discovered her sexuality with a young girl when she was twelve (SA Neptune=Asc, with tr Pluto square Sun, tr Jupiter conjunct Jupiter, and many more measurements).

She began to masturbate when she was eight (SA Mercury=Mars, Venus$_5$= Asc, with tr Uranus conjunct Venus). She continues masturbating three-four times daily, even in relationships and at age twenty-four.

It is very interesting to note that natal Pluto is conjunct Claudia's Midheaven, quintile her Ascendant. This Pluto-Midheaven position often corroborates exhibitionism, and Claudia tells her story in intelligent and detailed narrative on the Internet, on a special sexuality forum, for the world to read.

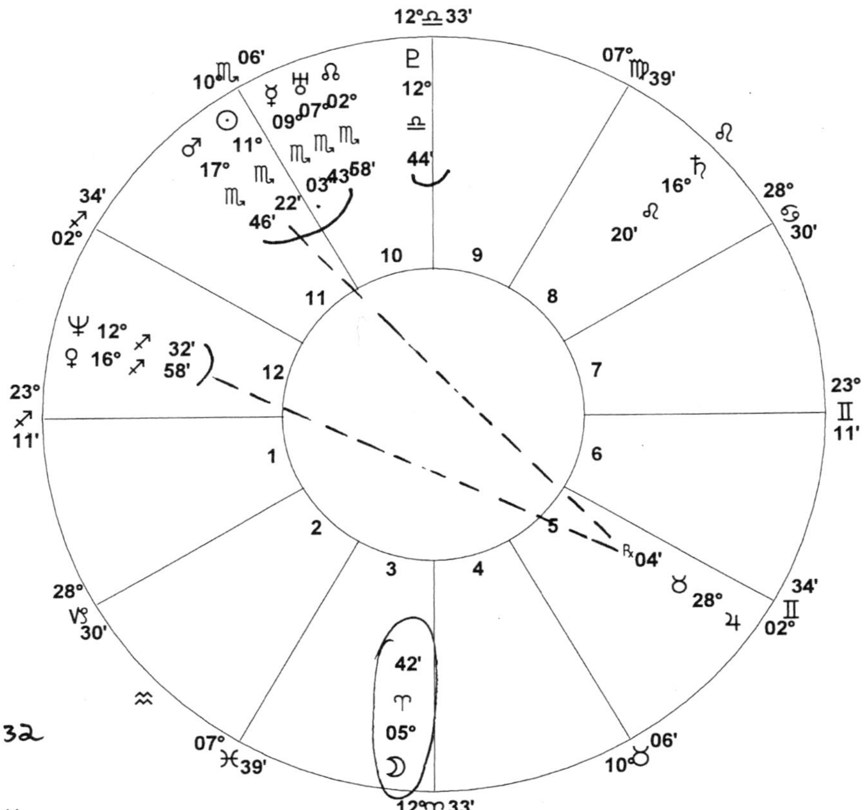

☽ 23♈32

♃ = ♆/♀, ♀/♅
♀ = ♆/A

		☉	☿	♀	♂	♃	♄	♅	♆	♇	☊	Mc
☉												
☿		☌a 02°19										
♀												
♂		☌a 06°23										
♃		q a 01°42										
♄		□a 04°58		△s 00°38	□s # 01°25							
♅	⊼a 02°01	☌s 03°39	☌s ∥ 01°20									
♆				☌s 04°26		q a 00°33	△s 03°49					
♇						⚼a 00°21	✱s 03°37		✱s 00°12			
☊			☌s 06°05	∠a 01°00				☌s 04°45				
Mc	☍s # 06°51					⚼a 00°31	✱a 03°47		✱s 00°01	☌a 00°11		
Asc			∠a 00°52	☌s 06°13				∠s 00°28		Qa 01°33		Qs 01°22

Chart 21
"Claudia"

Within this section of our discussion about hypersexuality, we must include two outstanding male examples: John F. Kennedy (May 29, 1917 at 3:00 P.M., EST in Brookline, Massachusetts) and Bill Clinton (August 19, 1946 at 8:51 A.M., CST in Hope, Arkansas).

Each has a Libra Ascendant, which very frequently puts Aquarius on the cusp of the 5th and Taurus on the cusp of the 8th, introducing the importance of Uranus and Venus, hypersexuality indeed.

Kennedy's $Uranus_5$ squares his stellium in the 8th (Mars, Mercury, Jupiter, Sun, and Venus). Venus rules the 8th. The Moon is square Venus.

Kennedy's (Sun in Gemini) nervous system (Uranus-Mercury square) is clearly caught up within the sexuality profile, propelling it for ego confirmation (Venus rules the Ascendant)

Clinton's $Uranus_5$ is smoothly trined by Jupiter. His $Venus_8$ is conjoined by Mars and Neptune (Mars-Neptune contacts promise charisma and allure), all in Libra at the Ascendant.

Orgasmic Difficulty/Dysfunction

The concern of difficulty with orgasm is particularly directed to females. This difficulty has long been within the awareness of relational sexuality, with medical references to the problem and to different solutions going back minimally 120 years. Early marketers of electric vibrators in the 1920s made little effort to camouflage their design for masturbation use in the female market; doctors offered female patients stimulation of many kinds to alleviate "female moods and dissipate stress."

It is rare for a man to have difficulty with orgasm in sex: his sexual organ is much more external and obvious than the female's, easily attracting touch and friction and responding easily, normally, to arousal. Literature for all of history speaks of the man's seed spewing forth. It was the man who made children; the woman just carried them. Men enjoyed sex; women didn't. Men explored their sexuality, with it becoming part of the conquest persona;

women were attendant to all this, often the victims. So much of this primal attitude exists still today in the prescriptions for male/female roles in Western society.

Times now are freer than ever before. Within the Information Age, information about sex abounds. People talk more freely about sexuality and sex in the most specific terms. Anxiety is alleviated by knowing; problems are solved through the dissemination of information. Just look how homosexuality has "come out of the closet" within the last generation! It has practically ceased to be a problem for most individuals, for society in general, whereas not so long ago it was classed as a mental disorder, a disease, by the medical profession.

Communication about sexuality in schools and colleges, and in the public media has brought so much vitally important information about sex to the public. Techniques of sexual expression; what to expect; what is possible; how to appreciate our drives, all this is "out there" for learning and discussion. Similarly, communication between two people is vitally important in the sharing of needs, the focusing of expectations to afford the beginnings of intimacy, leading to love and allowing sexuality to bloom harmoniously and meaningfully.

Yet, female orgasmic response *in relationship* is still frequently problematic. In the light of public media depictions of the sexual woman, any dysfunction is embarrassing. With men still having a lot to learn about sexuality, especially from the female's perspective, the male easily takes orgasmic shortfall by the woman as *criticism:* it's his fault, nothing he does works; he is less the man. The female was once called "frigid" when orgasm was not forthcoming to crown the sex act; now she is "not with the program" or "she has a problem," but down deep, the male suspects it is somehow "his fault." Often, the woman will displace her guilt onto the male in the form of criticism.

Interestingly, a woman who has orgasmic difficulty in relationship usually has no problem at all privately in masturbation. Almost invariably, the problem is not sexual at all, but a *relationship concern* that is causing difficulties (or some trauma from early development involving abuse or severely unsatisfactory relationship). And the presence of this relationship concern is an impediment to the larger profile of intimacy, as we have been studying together.

The content of the fantasy used in private erotic times[36] is often very important for its symbolism. For the woman, images of possession and compulsion or exhibitionism, for example, are usually symbolic statements of being forced to know that one is loved, desired, and cherished; this knowledge—trusting it—allows the full sexual response. No one else is in the way.[37]

The female difficulty is often due to a lack of trust of herself, the relationship partner, or the process. Amazingly, even with all the information about sexuality available, operational anatomical knowledge is still often lacking in the woman, very often in the man; knowledge of the process of clitoral stimulation, patience, time, mental constructs, loving closeness, etc. is not put into play. The difficulty emerges through the matrix of self-worth concerns, lovability issues, parental influence (including their modeling), and the idealized focus within masturbation success. This is why outstanding therapies for dysfunction involve bringing the reliable masturbatory technique into the dyadic relationship, to transfer/introduce the reliable solo response into the relationship process. We can see that this step of trust and sharing is part of building the confidence required by intimacy; both partners would certainly be developing in the same direction here.

Our objective here is to show how such difficulty with orgasm may be suggested in the female horoscope, opening up the topic for discussion and remediation.

Chart 22: "Janet"

"Janet's" horoscope (p. 130) shows that Pluto rules the 5th House, is in the 2nd House, and is squared by Saturn, normally a most debilitating aspect. In

---

36 And the fantasy is usually singular and repeated time and time again. It has arousal predictability.

37 Please see the detailed discussion in Tyl, *Synthesis & Counseling in Astrology*, 553–626.

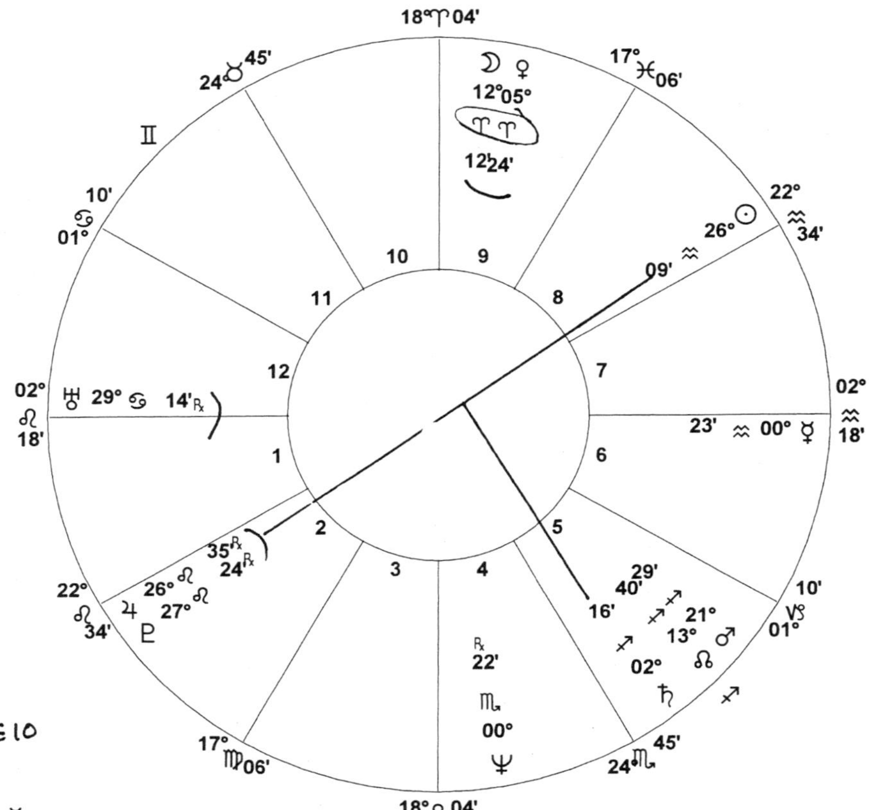

☽ 19♓10

AP=♄/♅

	☽	☉	☿	♀	♂	♃	♄	♅	♆	♇	☊	Mc
☉	∠s 01°03											
☿	Qa 00°12											
♀	☌s 06°47											
♂												
♃	⚻s 00°37	☍a # 00°26			△a 05°06							
♄		□a 06°08	⚹a ∥ 01°53	△s 03°08		□s 05°41						
♅			☍s 01°09				△s 03°02					
♆		△a 04°13	□s 00°02			⚹s 03°47		□s 01°08				
♇	⚻a 00°13	☍a 01°16			△a # 05°56	☌s 00°49	□s 04°52		⚹s 02°57			
☊	△a 01°28	Qs 00°29	∠s 01°44		∥			⚻s 00°34	∠s 01°42	#		
Mc	☌s 05°52				△a 03°25		⚻s 00°47				△s 04°24	
Asc			☍s # 01°55	△a 03°06			△s 00°02	☌s 03°04	□s 01°56			

Chart 22

"Janet"

turn, Pluto opposes the Sun (a smothering of selfhood, the blanket over a hand grenade). It is interesting to note that Saturn in the 5th rules the 6th, which is the twelfth House dynamic of the 7th, suggesting that a sexual difficulty would undermine relationship strongly.

Saturn squares the Sun, ruler of the self-worth 2nd.

There is this very heavy T-Square Jupiter-Pluto opposing the Sun, with Saturn squaring the axis, involving three Houses of the key Succedent Grand Cross.

The positive dimensions surrounding the problem are the comfortable Venus factor (note its conjunction with the Moon), ruling the 11th (she feels well loved); the pride of the Leo ascendant, attacked by Saturn and Pluto, but pushed to prevail through Uranus conjunct the Ascendant; AP=Saturn/Uranus promising a break from the old (the early home life influences) and the adoption of the new, the individually fashioned life; the very positive Pluto=Sun/Jupiter, promising great good fortune through self-application.

Another interesting feature here is the ego emphasis (reigning need to be *numero uno*) that will go a long way to propel Janet thorough any problem, and the Venus in Aries as well. Venus in Aries carries with it a flirtatiousness, a testing of others to see if one is appreciated, desired—not for sexual fulfillment but for ego confidence.

Chart 23: "Ingrid"

"Ingrid" (p. 132) shows Venus in Aries as well, augmented by Jupiter; i.e., there should be exaggerated flirtatiousness or contact with others to see what kind of effect she will have. Again, we see the Venus tie with the Moon, particularly elevated in Libra.

But look at the tremendous accentuation of the 2nd–8th House axis, especially the Saturn quindecile with Pluto, ruler of the 11th and Pluto's conjunction with Uranus, ruler of the 2nd. Saturn, here under high developmental tension, rules the Ascendant.

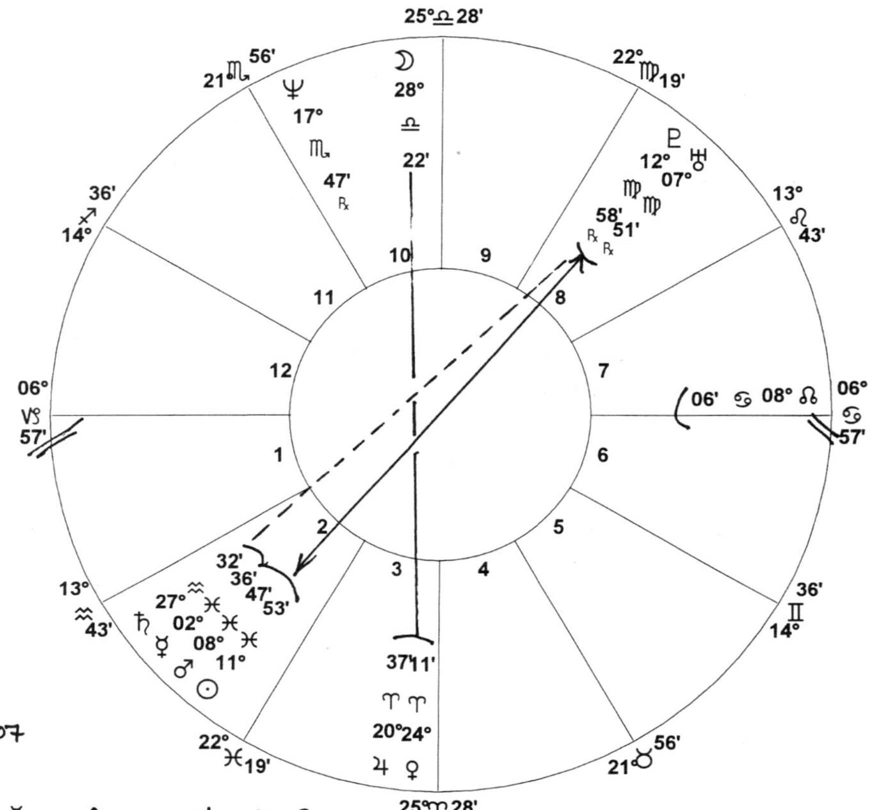

☽ 5♌07

	☽	☉	☿	♀	♂	♃	♄	♅	♆	♇	☊	Mc
☉	⚼s∥ 01°29											
☿	△a 04°14											
♀	☍s 04°11											
♂		☌s 03°06	☌a 06°11	∠s# 00°23								
♃	#	#		☌s 03°34								
♄	△s 00°50		☌s∥ 05°04	✶a 03°21								
♅		☍s 04°02	☍a 05°15	⚼s∥ 01°19	☍s# 00°56	⚼a 02°14						
♆		△a 05°54						Qa 02°04				
♇	∠s 00°24	☍a 01°04			☍a 04°10		q a 00°26	☌s 05°06				
☊		△s 03°47	△a 05°30	Qa 01°56	△s 00°41			✶a 00°15				
Mc	☌a 02°54	⚼a 01°25		☍s# 01°17	⚼s∥ 01°40	☍s 04°51	△a 02°04	#		∠a 02°30		
Asc					✶a 01°50			△a 00°54			☍a# 01°09	Qs 00°31

Asc=☉/☽, ☽/♇
AP=♀/♅

Chart 23

"Ingrid"

The hemisphere emphasis is to the North, unfinished business in the early home, and the Nodal axis is conjunct the horizon. The Moon semi-square with Pluto echoes this. The emphasis on the mother relationship is enormous.

Note that the sensitive Pisces Sun, ruler of the 8th House, is under great tension with Mars, Uranus, and Pluto.

Even though the Venus, ruler of the 5th, is in comfortable position, we see the self-worth crisis, the lovability crisis, the pronounced mother situation; overall, a "blanket over her hand grenade." We can easily suspect a problem with giving and receiving love, with sexual activity.

Ingrid is completely estranged from her mother; "I don't love my family," she says in a matter-of-fact way.

Ingrid has great difficulty with sexual response in relationship, and has been to a psychotherapist. She works as a masseuse/prostitute. Her main enjoyment from her work is that she can please the men and that they think she is magnificent (Jupiter-Venus in Aries).

Ingrid has recently met a man through her work who truly loves her, and through their relationship she is trying to gain self-respect and confidence in herself, trust in him, create intimacy, a change of work direction, and relationship fulfillment (tr Pluto square her Sun).

The extraordinarily clear and dramatic case of Marilyn Monroe bears repeating here (June 1, 1926 at 9:30 A.M., PST in Los Angeles, California): a classic Saturn$_{Rx}$ complex drives the entire horoscope. Venus operates in overcompensation in Aries at the Midheaven, ruling the Midheaven! Jupiter rules her 5th and is squared by the very difficult Saturn$_{Rx}$ and opposed by Neptune, ruling the 8th, also squared by Saturn$_{Rx}$! Marilyn suffered a life of complete sexual response dysfunction, well annotated in biographies and the papers of her psychotherapist (W. Hugh Missildine; see Steinem, *Marilyn*).[38]

---

38 See many references and studies of Monroe's horoscope in Tyl, *Synthesis & Counseling in Astrology*, especially 602–614.

In a case of near astral twins, the woman and the man having a Uranus-Venus conjunction in Taurus, *with Venus retrograde*, each opposed by the Moon in Scorpio, two manifestations occur: the woman is orgasmically dysfunctional because of fears grounded in early development and sexual trauma, now transferred into difficult relationship concerns, withdrawing for protection; the man, fearing that he may not be attractive and may be sexually rejectable, is compelled to prove himself sexually, constantly, making conquests continuously, actually keeping score, wearing all this as a badge of masculinity. The counterpoint of Venus retrogradation speaks of difficulty, a second agenda, individually wrought in their life.

Impotence

Men are loath to admit that they have a sexual problem, concern, or anxiety. Any such shortcoming diminishes them in the eyes of enormous societal emphasis on masculine importance, for the man to be strong, potent. Stories, pictures, and discussions—throughout the public media from academia to pornography—deal with the size of the penis and its value to women. In the main, these "studies" are fanciful, very often intimidating, and, I should suggest, hurtful within the stream of sexuality information available today.

Men's sensitivity about their virility keeps them from seeking medical advice, especially with reference to symptoms that might suggest erectile difficulty, prostate gland conditions (including cancer), etc. Men are supposed to be invulnerable, indestructible, and eternally enduring when it comes to sex. When I have inquired about a client getting a sexually specific check-up from a urologist, I have been told many, many times, "No; I don't want to know."

But the fact remains that the beginning of a loss of erectile strength and vitality, urination frequency and urgency are signs of aging and/or several diseases, the most important of which are related to the prostate gland or to the testicles. While impotence can be brought about at any age by psychological and developmental concerns, treatment of prostate or testicular conditions presents this side effect quite clearly. Men fear this, do not get medical attention, the condition worsens, anxiety spills over into other relational areas of life, the support bond suffers in the marriage. Intimacy has been challenged and fractured. Criticism, rejection, abandonment.

Particular vulnerability to prostatic, testicular, or gastro-intestinal weakness is suggested in the male horoscope through hard measurements involving Pluto, often with Saturn and/or Neptune, the ruling planet of the 12th House, the Sun, and Ascendant.[39] For our discussion here, *we must be alert to these symbologies manifesting as well in sexual anxieties about penis size, sex drive, and/or impotence.*

At the same time, astrologers must be aware of therapeutic counsel in cases of impotence. A visit to any urologist's office and some study in the library or on the Internet can provide important information about the use of vacuum erection devices (pumps) and the pill trademarked Viagra. But even without an erection—when one gets past the embarrassment, i.e., when one explores the grace of intimacy—sexual response occurs to orgasm with or without ejaculation, led by the mind and a very special set of nerve networks. Impotence is not the end of the road of sexual expression by any means!

The Mind

The most sensitive and powerful sexual organ is the mind. The mind conceives, desires, plans, guides, communicates, evaluates, and remembers all that is connected with sexuality. When there is underachievement or dysfunction, the mind cleverly (instinctively) explains it often at the expense of the other person, protecting (aggrandizing) ego as best it can. Schemes of criticism and/or rejection can be concocted *before the other person* criticizes or rejects. Complicated, years-long, self-protecting postures and behaviors can be put into the life, fomenting battle after battle between two people in a

39 Please see Tyl, *The Astrological Timing of Critical Illness*, for full discussion of these conditions with many examples.

relationship deficient sexually. People often make themselves unattractive (overweight, grooming, rudeness, etc.) in order not to face the challenge and eventual embarrassment of relationship and poor sexual functioning.

Of course these problems develop out of the early homelife concerns we have studied in many cases in this book. It is in the nakedness of sexuality that they become urgently focused in frustration and fear.

The mind takes deep desire and frustration to symbolic levels (as in dreams) to be satisfied in private eroticism. Inspection of sexual fantasy very often tells an important emotional story: the male fantasy of two women sexually engaged as he watches or another man pleasing his own wife can suggest his extreme desire to see the woman fulfilled, perhaps warding off his fear that he is less than capable, someone else is doing it for me and I can enjoy that fact, even take credit for it. The female fantasy content often involves being possessed or coerced to prove to herself that she is intensely desirable, or if with another woman, often the "other" woman is simply the self in idealized form, thinner, blonder, freer, etc. It is simply getting very close to the idealized self-image.

The mind makes sex happen: sending the signal to the penis to become erect (or not to); the mind gives the signal for the female to allow sexual activity (or not to). Within guilt patterns perhaps, the mind can induce premature ejaculation by the male as an escape from the act, from the relationship. The mind can create orgasmic pretense by the woman in order to satisfy male expectations, albeit falsely. Private fantasy life fans the fires of unfulfillment, calling attention intensely to the relationship difficulties focused in relationship.

All of this activity leads sooner or later to loneliness, to incompleteness. There is no relationship left, little room or traffic for trust, no development of intimacy. We do not feel we are acceptable or understood; a feeling of emptiness eats away at the person *who doubts his/her own lovableness* (and we have learned clearly and dramatically that this dimension within the Succedent Grand Cross is focused chiefly through the 11th House and it significator).

One of the symptoms of depression is a loss of sexual interest. The mind is being diverted from the normal spectrum of interests. The mind can conceive the fantastic or the excessive in times of mania, can create complex requirements for sexual fulfillment. The mind can allow love projection upon several "others" simultaneously. The mind can internalize religious, peer group, or parental standards obsessively, affecting sexual expression strongly.

The mind can be dulled by alcohol, making erection less than ideal or actually impossible for the male, making sex sloppy and unattractive for the woman. Alcohol can then become a way *to avoid* sexual contact; it can be rationalized as a way to unwind from a hard day's work, but it is designed to mask avoidance of the situation in which criticism (implicit or explicit) will be encountered. Rejection will then somehow avoid that level of hurt; abandonment can be just around the corner, with the problems being repeated similarly in the next relationship.

We must understand that the mind uses all we learn, know, and experience. The mind uses this vastness to transmit our personalized energy into our work to fulfill our reigning need and our subsidiary needs. The mind has internalized all the dynamics of societal expectations, family modeling, and the press of individual needs. The mind leads us into functioning identity. Perhaps this is the reason that Mercury is always so close to the Sun.

Mercury, its Sign and House condition, and the 3rd House (the mindset) suggest the mind's orientation within all we do, of course, *including sexuality*. Sex-scandalized preacher Jimmy Swaggart (March 15, 1935 at 1:35 A.M., CST in Ferriday, Louisiana) has his Mercury in Aquarius (i.e., he needs to think in ways of social service; in avant garde ways), squared by Jupiter (that need is augmented, possibly colored by religion, philosophy), ruling the 7th, with Neptune, the ruler of the 3rd, peregrine. This Neptune colors the mindset, adding a fantasy dimension to it, a camouflage, as the very strong sexuality profile is expressed [Venuss opposed by Mars and squared by Pluto).

Sex-scandalized President Bill Clinton has Mercury in Leo (the need to express thought with ego theatricality) conjoined Pluto (mega-thoughts, an extreme measure), and his Jupiter, ruling his 3rd, trines (easy flow) *Uranus ruling his 5th*. His Venus ruling the 8th is conjoined Mars and rules his Ascendant. An extremely powerful sexual profile is the center of his identity and his mind knows it, uses it dramatically, egocentrically.

It is interesting indeed that Swaggart and Clinton both have Mercury conjunct Saturn—far from being suppressed in these specially developed people, the mind is turned to serve ambition powerfully.

John F. Kennedy had his Mercury in Taurus (the plan for security) in the 8th, squared by Uranus, ruler of his 5th. His 3rd was ruled by Jupiter, *conjunct Mercury in the 8th*. The Uranian contact with Mercury introduces strongly consideration of the nervous system; Jupiter augments it. Sex was tied strongly to Kennedy's nervous system, its poise, and his sense of ego security. His Pluto, ruling his 2nd, was peregrine; I think he was always concerned about being the son his father wanted him to be (in the place of his older, dead brother; Saturn_4-Neptune conjunction in the 10th) and sex was strongly tied to his self-evaluation and measure of personal security vis-à-vis others (stellium in the 8th).

Marlene Dietrich (Dec 27, 1901 at 9:15 P.M., CET in Berlin, Germany), had her Mercury in Capricorn (a sharp, strategic turn of mind) at the 5th cusp quindecile Pluto, itself trine Venus, ruler of the 3rd ; Mercury was opposed by Neptune, ruler of her 8th. Her thinking was obsessively ambitious and conquest-driven into a secret bisexual world [Neptune=Venus/Node=AP].

Music-dance-sex marketer Madonna (August 16, 1958 at 7:05 A.M., EST in Bay City, Michigan) has her $\text{Mercury}_{\text{Rx}}$ in Virgo in the 12th conjoined with Pluto, ruler of her 3rd. There is conflict in her sexuality profile: Saturn_5 trine the Sun (easy flow, a strategy/coercion overtone) and Mars_8 is squared by Uranus (great intensity). This conflict is reflected in the retrogradation counterpoint of Mercury, and in the Neptune square with Venus.

Princess Diana (July 1, 1961 at 7:45 P.M., GMD in Sandringham, England) had a strong sexuality profile with Venus in Taurus in the 5th and ruling that House, squared by Uranus in the 8th. The Moon ruling the 8th was opposed by Uranus. Her Mercury$_{Rx}$ was conjoined the Sun and quindecile to the Ascendant, suggesting at her core an obsessive, contrapuntal agenda about emotional security within an expected or prescribed ideal (Sun-Mercury conjunction; Jupiter$_{A}$ squared by Neptune), probably most debilitating, suppressing of Self.

"Alfred" (p. 124), has Mercury$_{Rx}$ in Pisces; the mind is in an emotional swoon, in the 8th, ruling the 11th *and* the 2nd. That Mercury is opposed by Uranus. The nervous system, the swoon, the idealization fantasies (Water Grand Trine) all work overtime to fulfill the needs of Venus in Aries, ruling the 3rd, being appreciated, loved, respected; a world of high-activity solo-sex.

Abuse

Sexual abuse occurs much more often than we generally know. Recent research reports state that there were 800,000 child abuse cases in the United States in 1999. That's more than 2,000 per day (!); over thirty years, say, the age spectrum of an astrologer's clientele, there could have been more than 24,000,000 cases reported.

The astrologer will too often uncover sexual abuse suffered by the client. The horoscope will not say "sexual abuse" in some specific symbolic formula, but it will suggest a precocious sexual time in life, usually before age ten (I have seen cases of child abuse starting so early and, incredibly, lasting as a routine into the early twenties!). Seeing an "attack" by Arc or transit to Venus or the ruler of the 5th, or to the Sun/Moon midpoint, by Pluto or Saturn, usually with a Neptune contact somehow with an Angle (early ego "wipe out"), the astrologer *asks a question about the time period:* "May I ask you please, was there any trauma at age five, perhaps in the late summer?" A question like this opens the door very easily or, should there not have been any abuse, the question can be passed over smoothly, going right on with the consultation with some other event that will be introduced by the client to fulfill the guideline suggestions of the measurements. The most important key here in such an instance is to determine *what the client can tell you she or he has carried forward from that time into later years.*

Chart 24: "Patty"

Horoscope 24 belongs to "Patty."

- The Hemisphere emphasis is to the North, suggesting unfinished business in the early home.
- Focusing on the sexual profile: the ruler of the 5th, Uranus is opposed Mars, ruler of the 7th, suggesting much anxiety and lack of trust within relationships, possibly coming from sexual issues.
- In the 5th we see Venus and Mercury in "idealistic" conjunction[40] opposed Pluto, ruler of the 2nd, and *quindecile* the Node. Here is a demanding and emphatic suggestion of the mother within 5th House affairs, relating to 2nd House concerns. Venus also rules the 8th.
- The Moon—seeking a mother-symbol echo here—rules the parental 10th, is exactly squared by Neptune, and is *quindecile the Midheaven!*
- Additionally, Pluto=Sun/Moon, with the Sun-Moon relationship involving the two parents as well as Patty's own relationships with the world, under stress through $Mars_7$ opposed Uranus.
- And finally, focused on this emerging issue, we have another midpoint picture, a difficult one, Pluto=Saturn/Asc: "violent upset, deep anguish, being put down by others."

Read Patty's own words:

> I too am a survivor of childhood sexual abuse, and for years I lived in a state of emotional numbness with recurrent seasonal (winter) depressions that often incapacitated me. Noel amazed me in my consultation with him last May when, within the first three minutes of our conversation, he said he saw "mother" written all over my

---

40 Please see "Idealism," Tyl, *Synthesis & Counseling in Astrology*, 105–112.

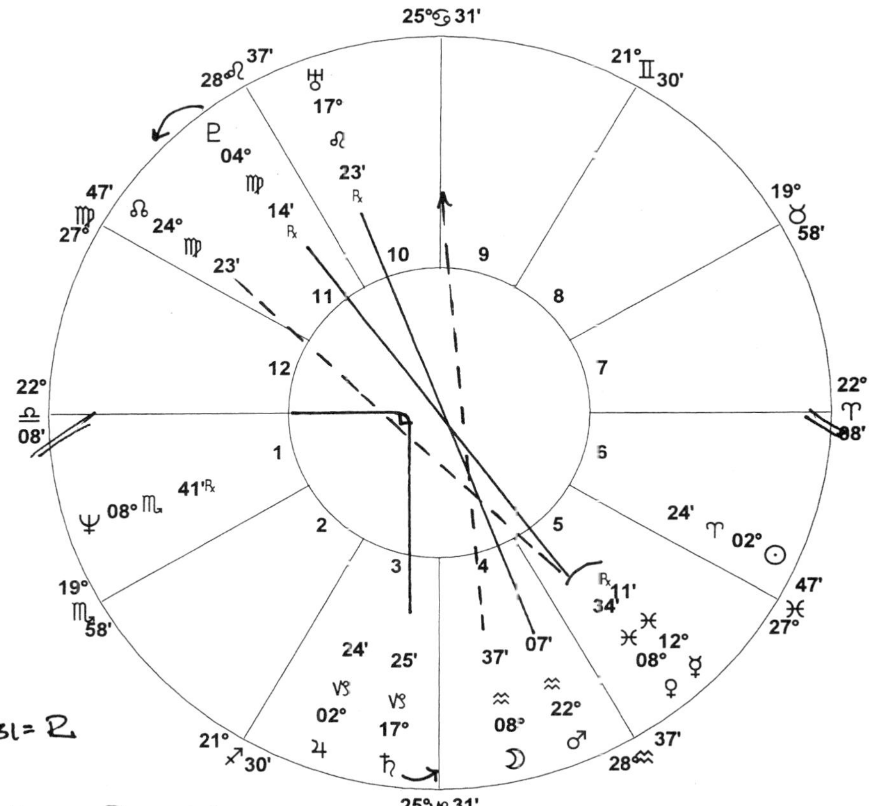

☽ 5♓31 = ♇

♇ = ♄/A

☉		☉										
☿			☿									
♀			♂a 03°37	♀								
♂	‖				♂							
♃		□s 00°00	Qs 02°13			♃						
♄							♄					
♅		⚼s 00°02			☍s 04°44	⚼s 00°01	⊼s 00°02	♅				
♆	□a 00°04		△a 03°30	△a 00°06					♆			
♇		⊼a 01°49		☍s 04°21		△a 01°50	⚼a ∦ 01°49			♇		
☊	⚼a 00°46			q a 00°48	⊼a 02°16				∠a 00°42		☊	
Mc	q s 01°54		⚼a 01°40	⚼s 01°57			∦			‖	✱s 01°08	Mc
Asc				⚼a ‖ 01°27	△s 00°01	Qs 01°44	□s 04°43					□s 03°23 Asc

Chart 24

"Patty"

> chart. My mother was my abuser. Noel was able to see from my chart specifics about the abuse it took me years of therapy to uncover.
>
> . . . I've had to deal with extreme emotional sensitivity and anxiety all my life. My defense was always to dissociate and go numb inside. I remember during my first two years of therapy feeling far away, almost out-of-body, whenever I talked about my feelings with my therapist. It was as if I was up by the ceiling in the corner of the room looking down on myself, totally detached from my emotions. [This is the ultimate defense against terrible hurt: dissociation, even the creation of other personalities, to assimilate somehow the enormous trauma of abuse.]
>
> After years of therapy, I was able to get my depressions under control and begin coming out of my emotional isolation. I need very much to be around and relate to people [the Moon in Aquarius and the Libra Ascendant, with Mars$_7$ trine the Ascendant . . . combating the Uranus opposition with Mars$_7$], but all the "unfinished business" from my childhood has made it difficult for me to relate to people in the way I need to in order to thrive.

In our consultation, I just mentioned the word "mother" to Patty, and she replied that her mother had sexually abused her. The association of word and abuse experience was immediate. We discussed this softly for a moment, timing it to about the age span of four to eight [SA Pluto=Venus with Saturn=MC]. I suggested that the abuse was anal (typically punitive enemas), led by the natal Pluto opposition to the Sun/Moon midpoint in the 5th House.

Patty's mother was mentally ill. Patty was moved away from her mother at age thirteen, when tr Uranus came to her Ascendant and tr Saturn squared her Sun simultaneously.

Finally, after much therapy, Patty manages this difficult issue very well. Her mind had been hurt so by it all: Mercury$_{Rx}$ in vulnerable Pisces conjunct Venus (idealized expectations, shocked by the terrible hurt of reality) opposed in extremism by Pluto.

Chart 25: "Louise"

"Louise's" horoscope (p. 145) presents seven observations that strongly suggest difficulty in the sexual area, with sharp reference to mother and father, exacerbated through Arc reference at a very early age [Asc=Uranus at age four with tr Pluto opposed Sun].

- Northern Hemisphere emphasis (indicated by the retrogradation pattern in the Southern Hemisphere).
- Mars, ruler of the 5th, quindecile with Pluto$_{12}$ (always a statement of severity, as we have seen).
- Mercury$_{10, 7}$ quindecile the Node (mother).
- Saturn$_{Rx}$ (father) ruler of her self-worth 2nd, squared by Neptune$_4$.
- Venus$_{11}$ opposed by Neptune$_4$.
- Moon in Scorpio, ruling the 8th, is in the 12th.
- Sun peregrine, i.e., dissociated.

Read Louise's own words, focused on the dissociation complex (Sun) defending against sexual abuse:

> I have sexual abuse in my history. I was diagnosed in 1989 with what is now called Dissociate Identity Disorder. The old term for it was MPD [Multiple Personality Disorder]: sexual trauma sets up the nervous system to defend against everything at all times, especially when multiple family members are involved and there's no one to trust in order to model a healthy Self. Dissociation results from splitting off the intolerable pain of the memory. Adult behaviors such as unstable relationships, an identity established by circumstance rather than by Self, and wildly fluctuating moods are the rule.
>
> When I was sick with DID, I owned two wardrobes, had two body sizes complete with radical hairstyle changes. One personality had certain allergies and the other didn't. One personality was dyslexic, had undiagnosed vision problems and could not read without great

> difficulty, and the other had 20/20 vision and read with the comprehension of a college graduate while in high school.
>
> The amazing thing about me during my illness is that I managed to put myself through college, graduating with honors [Sun rules the 8th], marry, successfully raise a child and start and run my own business [now national in scope]. . . . I was what is termed a "high functioning" dissociative. It took an amazing, gifted psychologist trained in treating dissociative disorders to bring me to myself after seven painful years of uncovering the traumas.

Clearly in Louise's horoscope, the mother issue is enormous with Mercury, a parental ruler exactly *quindecile* the Node. Then there is Saturn$_{Rx}$ square the axis of Venus-Neptune, in the parental axis. Finally, *Mars*$_{5}$ *is quindecile Pluto, ruler of the 12th.*

Louise was ritually abused by her family who were Satanists deeply involved with occult practices. Her urethra and colon were severely damaged. The abuse began at age four and lasted to age eleven. The victimization syndrome extended into her marriage. Her first husband was deeply involved in morbid photography, her second husband turned out to be a pedophile, apprehended by the police.

Louise continues:

> In 1989 [accumulated semisquare Solar Arc, with tr Saturn conjunct the Sun/Moon midpoint] I divorced myself from my mother.
>
> . . . I consider myself the poster child of horrid relationships. Although I've matured over the years, relating for me is not a given [Mercury rules the 7th, a carry over of tensions from Mercury's Node connection, with Uranus in the 7th sesquiquadrate with Mars]. You know a lot about me, Noel, and I give you permission to "go for it." I would appreciate the subject of sexual abuse discussed openly, as the abuse I suffered at age four onward is the root of my inability to relate comfortably.

Louise is a keenly intelligent woman. Her Mercury in Aquarius, offering her experience to help others, is trined by Jupiter at the Midheaven.

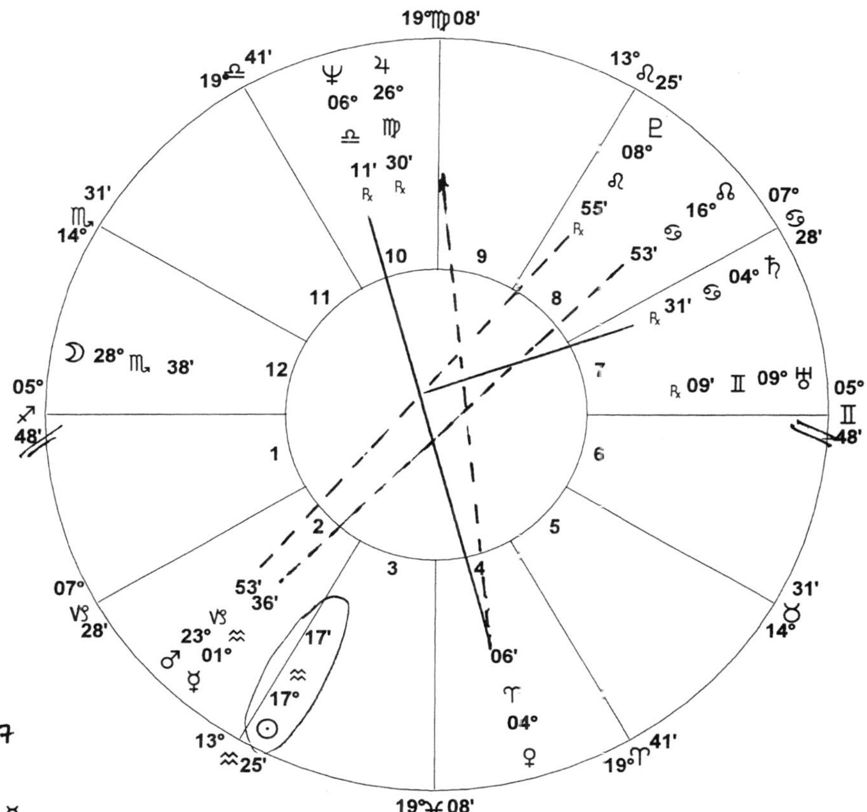

	☽ 7♑57	☉	☿	♀	♂	♃	♄	♅	♆	♇	☊	Mc
☉	∥											
☿	✱a 02°58											
♀	Δa 05°28	∠a 01°49	✱a 02°30									
♂			∥	Qa 01°47								
♃	✱s 02°08		Δs 05°06	∥	Δa 02°37							
♄		⚻a 02°15		□a 00°25	∦							
♅			∦		⚻a∦ 00°16		∥					
♆			Δa 04°35	☍a 02°05			□s 01°40	Δs 02°57				
♇				Δa 04°49	q a 00°02			✱s 00°14	✱a 02°44			
☊		⊼s 00°24	q a 00°17		∦	Qs 02°23	∥	∥				
Mc		⊼s 01°52		q s 00°02	Δa 04°44						✱s 02°16	
Asc		Qs 00°31	∥	Δs 01°42	∥		⊼s 01°17	☍a∦ 03°21	✱a 00°23	Δa 03°07		

Chart 25

"Louise"

General Astrological Considerations

The subject of sexuality is vast. It is within the sexuality profile that we find developmental problems focusing themselves most vividly, as gender expectations set by society and individual potentials present themselves for confirmation, alone and in relationship. If there is a self-worth concern, an anxiety about being lovable, there will be to one degree or another difficulty or awkwardness with giving love. This immediately sets up difficulty with relating.

Without self-confidence, there is little trust possible of someone else. The fears of criticism, rejection, and abandonment, the enemies of intimacy, endure. Sexual problems in relationship make matters worse. Communication to heal these tensions usually evaporates—everything is swept under the rug, only to appear as tensions in other dimensions of interaction. Recall please our study of the negative anima and negative animus projections, chapter 3.

Several measurement specifics, highly supported empirically, can add to illumination of the sexuality profile and help discussion during astrological consultation:

Venus in the 12th House often corresponds to a "private sense of beauty," hard to fulfill, hard to please. The aesthetic and emotional needs are privately protected within the accumulation of all that society says one should expect from relationship. The privacy of it all can make sexual fulfillment difficult. Adjustment of the idealization will be important to freeing up sexual expression, to bringing greater values to reality.

We have seen many cases of Venus retrograde. This is a very sensitive signification: the retrogradation introduces a counterpoint, a second agenda, a second or undercurrent line of emotional need-reasoning. Venus retrograde may register as debilitation in emotional fulfillment and/or sexual dysfunction. The "other" considerations or frustrations must be discussed: *"There is a suggestion here that there is more to this problem than we are talking about so far. What other concerns do you think are tied closely to this situation? What is really getting in the way?"* Venus House reference(s) by rulership may be very helpful in guiding the discussion into developmental experiences in the past.

Venus in Capricorn curiously suggests a delay in the maturing of relational values. There can be an apparent coldness, a methodical, clock-like way about the sexual process (Capricorn in general as well).

Venus in Aries has been present in many of our example cases. It connotes a kind of flirtatious nature that "tests" even casual acquaintances to see if one is attractive, desired. It is not necessarily an invitation to or readiness for sex; it is a kind of marketing survey for the emotions. Marilyn Monroe had Venus in Aries, Venus ruling her Midheaven.

With Saturn in the 11th, there is a tremendous need for love, for feeling valuable. This is not a simplistic suggestion; it is a deeply significant core-concern to the person and drives many activities in life development. It opens up a long list of vulnerabilities.

When Uranus is in the 11th, the expectation of love and attention is consciously keen and needs to be intensely, demonstratively, and immediately served. The partner must suit these guidelines, or there is no relationship harmony.

Uranus oriental (rising last of all the other planets before the Sun rises in clockwise motion) suggests adventure and daring as an important key to life expression, and will relate obviously to the sexuality profile if the ties are there appropriately.

Saturn-Venus aspects can introduce constrained emotional expression, possible sexual dysfunction, especially in the female; excessive sexual expression for ambition and ego reinforcement by the male; a conspicuous age difference in relationship, with the concomitant psychodynamic identification with parent figures, or constrained sexual expression.

Neptune configured in strong aspect with the Sun or the Moon, with Venus or Mercury, brings a sense of suppression or camouflage to sexuality, often when the 5th and/or the 8th House is involved by rulership or tenancy. If suppression does not fit the general synthesis of the horoscope or the client's reality, Neptune may simply refer to something else than that which is obvious, i.e., something is other than it seems wherever Neptune is located or where Neptune rules.

In the 7th House, Neptune suggests that the preferred partner is most usually in need of or depends on the person's support, help, and leadership. The relationship may be a pretense, a mask, a substitute for some other need complex.

In a male horoscope, Neptune strongly keyed to the 5th and/or the 8th and involved in a strong, apparently debilitating aspect structure can suggest embarrassment and even depression about genital size, sexual performance, or indeed, acute or chronic impotence. As well, Neptune in the 4th, the twelfth dynamic of the 5th, can figure strongly to vulnerability in the sexuality profile that, with age, may manifest as impotence, usually related to early familial occurrences, learned attitudes, relationship demands, or illness.

There is no need here to extend our study into the psychodynamically complex worlds of sadomasochism, bondage, prostitution, body-piercing, etc. These conditions appear in sexual profiles to one degree or another in lives from the conventional to the exorbitantly avant-garde in society. They are specialized areas that the astrologer will gradually absorb in further study of the field of sexuality.[41]

Does Sex Die?

The press of hormones, the social drives, the relationship gambits are so strong, so urgent, so many. For many people, the process of development, especially where sexuality plays its enormous role, is bewildering, exhausting, filled with insecurity, loneliness, and fears. When sexuality "does not *work* as it should," people frequently allow themselves to become unattractive in order not to invite another relationship failure; they choose to live alone with broken confidence, avoiding criticism, rejection, or abandonment in relationship. They experience the pain of loneliness, the antithesis of relationship.

---

41 Please see Tyl, ed. *Sexuality in the Horoscope* for 355 pages of sexuality discussion and study.

Celebrated psychiatrist/author David Viscott presents this case boldly, poignantly: "Of all feelings, loneliness is the worst. To be lonely is to lack something that makes you feel complete. Sometimes it is another person. Sometimes it is a part of yourself you want desperately to know really exists, a higher view of yourself that gives your life meaning."[42]

There is always the refuge of fantasy and social pretense, of throwing oneself into work, responsibilities, all kinds of activities, and for those feeling this way within a marriage, fatigue and preoccupation easily become respectable excuses for nonrelating, for not even being at home.

Others express exhilaration, confidence, gregariousness, family joy, and pleasure. But is this reliably so? I have heard the most externally perfected individuals, with social accomplishments and status, speak in the *intimacy of the consultation* [please think what that phrase means] about "not wanting my husband to touch me or even get near me!" or "I've given up on my wife; sex is such a chore; she's not with it anyhow; we go through the motions about twice a year; if people only knew!"

I think the point here is that sexuality plays its role early on in the social development of gaining a relationship, the way our society says it is supposed to be. The hormones, peer pressure, societal prescriptions are powerful. We tend to repeat what our parents have established—and remember, in many cultures, marriages used to be/are still *arranged* by the parents—while our inner environment of individualized needs sometimes fights a painful war.

When the bubbles burst—the idealistic projections of the perfect mate, according to what we learned a perfect mate should be—the negative animus and anima expressions can turn the marriage to struggle and bitterness. Personal needs are reorganized into different hierarchical arrangement in their press for expression. Usually, sexuality is the first major area to suffer.

With the aging process, the hormonal intensity diminishes; familiarity (routine) can breed boredom and distance, if not contempt. Private eroticism

---

42 Viscott, page 22.

can either intensify to express the frustrated individual sexuality profile or it can diminish drastically in surrender to frustration.

Sex easily dies, but *sexuality hides.* Intimacy is no longer a consideration since the reality of criticism, rejections, and abandonment has been all too real for all too long. Unfortunately, this is so very much the human condition, unless informed, objective, loving, fair communication has constructed a glowing but lasting bubble (i.e., away from the Hollywood image).

Our society speaks the adage so frequently, "You really have to work at relationship." And this pragmatic truth almost always accompanies the discovery of sexual infidelity (itself an extraordinarily difficult issue within the natural expression of sexuality, when very close to half of all men and women in marriages do "cheat").

Sexuality hides itself in memories, in fantasies, in aesthetic expression, and in private moments of catharsis, as opportunities to confirm the self. But sexuality *can* come out of hiding; it *can* rekindle a kinder way of relating based more on togetherness than on self-fulfillment. Older people somehow learn to grow past bitterness. Age can bring objectification, mutual respect, and recognition—finally—of how much each of us needs another.

6

RELATIONSHIPS
The Patterns that Show Difficulty

Magazine articles focusing on marriage are filled with dramatic statistics, that one of every two marriages will end in divorce; that, in spite of the difficulty with marriage, 90 percent of Americans still do marry. The societal prescriptions for each of us to marry are so strong that marriage is deemed *necessary* within our scheme of development. Marriage is undeniably established as the key adult relationship.

Seventy-five percent of those divorced get married yet again! Then, 60 percent of the remarriages fail.[43]

The reason for all this failure is familiar to us in the scope of our study in this book. Despite our individual best efforts, something goes wrong so very often. Initially, blame can emerge out of shocked animus and anima projections: it is always the *other* person who develops some critical character flaw or craziness. This is the bubble bursting, the disappointment of those animus/anima projections, the incompatibility of individual need profiles, camouflaged in the fantasy of romance early in the relationship. Yet, until our last dying breath, we still think, "Someday I'll meet someone perfect; he/she will fit with all my wonderful expectations," and another bubble is created.

---

43 *Psychology Today* magazine, March/April 2000, page 57.

The great allure, we know, is the primal need not to be alone, to be *with* someone, not just for procreation, but for support as well, to help us grow and advance in ways and into directions we can not navigate for ourselves. We want to share our being, including our "secret Self" wherein our individual needs, including our sexual needs, are so deeply focused.

We long for intimacy, that state of confidence and trust that will not experience criticism as punishment, will not anticipate rejection or final abandonment. Certainly, intimacy presumes confrontations with developmental problems, allowing objective assimilation of what is learned through developmental tensions, leading to respect for individuation—all that which will allow unselfish respect for someone else fighting the same developmental struggle.

Intimacy and honesty go together, and circumspect patterns of behavior must be established *early* in the relationship to afford a smooth transition from the romantic focus of getting together initially to the working partnership that will endure. Conflict is inevitable, of course, but it can be diffused with various constructive coping mechanisms worked out in communication, *cradled in the embrace of intimacy*.

Ted Huston, PhD., Ecology and Psychology professor at the University of Texas at Austin, shares reports of his long-term study of marriages. He found that brief courtships do not allow realistic formation of relationship expectations. He found that many newlyweds are far from blissfully in love, that couples whose marriages begin in romantic bliss are particularly divorce-prone because such intensity is too hard to maintain; in other words, marriages that start out with less "Hollywood romance" usually have more promising futures.

Huston found that spouses in lackluster marriages are less divorce-prone, i.e., their marriages are less fulfilling to begin with, so there is no breakdown of idealism—the bubble isn't so fragile or unrealistic as to burst!

He found that the loss of love and affection, not the emergence of interpersonal issues, is what leads people to divorce.[44] This tells us that *there is a*

44 *Psychology Today* magazine, January/February 2000, page 60.

breakdown of intimacy; boredom and routined dullness emerge. This reveals the lack of *personal* fulfillment, and *that* is what leads to divorce.

Consultation

Here is the astrology of a divorce; it is "Julia" divorcing her husband. Recall the orientation to her horoscope (p. 26); her natal chart is reprinted here.

Facing Julia's natal chart is the chart for the time of consultation, chosen spontaneously by both of us, diverging from my practice of suggesting consultation appointments on the hour. This was a telephone consultation set for 7:30 A.M., MST at my location, 9:30 A.M. EST at hers.

Note that Consultation Chart Mars is *exactly square the midpoint of Julia's natal Sun and Moon* (2 Virgo 39). This alerts us that the consultation would probably be focused upon tension in a relationship, her marriage. As well, we see *CC Uranus conjunct Julia's Midheaven and her natal Uranus at 8 Virgo applying to conjunction with the CC 7th House cusp.* Three strong measurements spoke of marriage tension.

And that's what the consultation was for: Julia had decided to divorce her husband.

Now, become familiar with this combined presentation of Direct and Indirect Solar Arcs and major Transits in Julia's horoscope for a year's time (pp. 156–157.[45] Note the fourth and fifth columns: these columns show the SA activity (Ar), the "hits" made by the Secondary Progressed Moon (Pr), and the major transits in the fourth harmonic (Tr). The dates in the second column are precise for the computer, but we must recognize time-orb as we read the dates and think in terms of the *month* initially, instead of the exact date of partile [more specificity can often be determined through experience with transits and through Tertiary Progressions; see Tyl, *Solar Arcs.*].

The analytical comments written to the right, outside the boxed measurements, are keys for our discussion; it is how I prepare my worksheet before

45 Full explanation of such a dynamic SA-SP Moon-Transit Flow Chart is presented in Tyl, *Solar Arcs.*

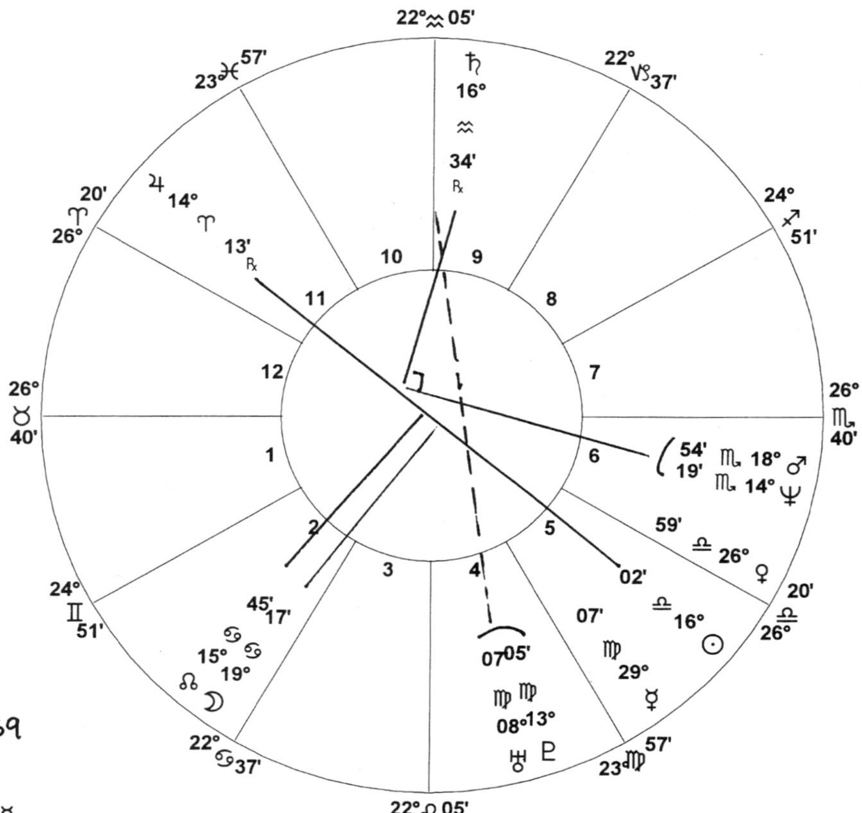

☽ 2♏39

	☽	☉	☿	♀	♂	♃	♄	♅	♆	♇	☊	Mc
☉	□s 03°15											
☿	Qs 02°10											
♀												
♂	△s 00°22											
♃	□s 05°03	☍s 01°49	q a 00°07									
♄		△a 00°32	⚼a 02°27		□s ‖ 02°21	✶s 02°20						
♅				‡	Qa 01°13							
♆	△s 04°57		∠a 00°13		☌s 04°35	⊼s 00°06	□a 02°14					
♇				∠a 01°06		⊼a 01°09		☌a 04°57	✶s 01°15			
☊	☌s ‖ 03°32	□s 00°17	Qs 01°21		△s 03°09	□s 01°32	⊼s 00°49		△a 01°26	✶a 02°41		
Mc				△a 04°54	□s 03°10		☌s 05°31	q a 01°03	‖			
Asc			△a 02°26	⊼a 00°18						‖		□a 04°36

Chart 4

"Julia"

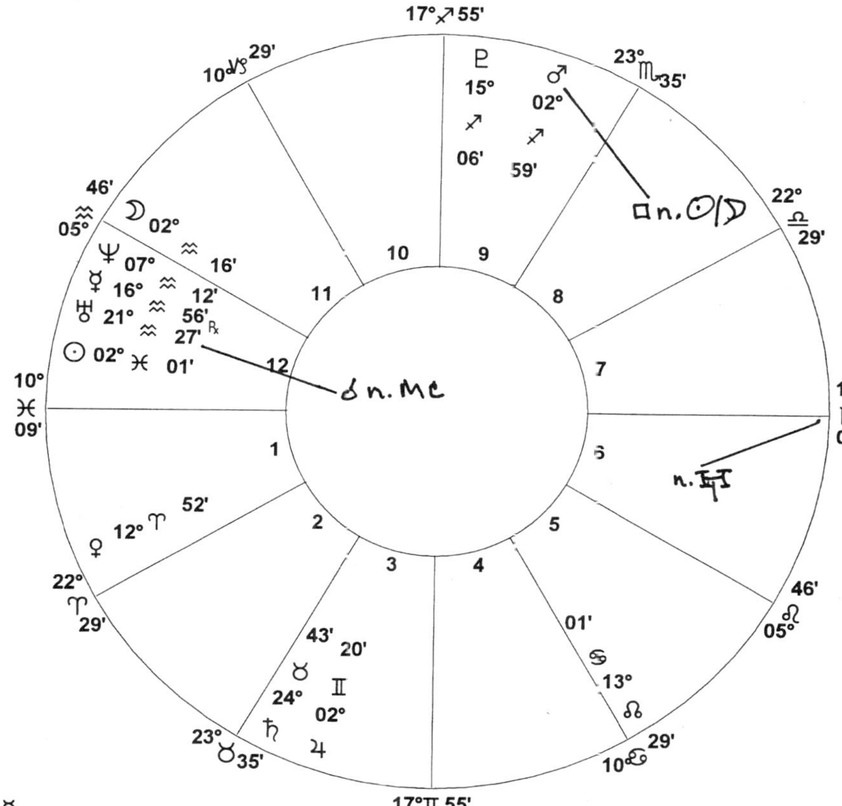

	☽	☉	☿	♀	♂	♃	♄	♅	♆	♇	☊	Mc
☉												
☿												
♀	Qs 01°24											
♂	✶a 00°43	□a 00°58	Qa 01°56									
♃	△a 00°04	□a 00°19			☍s ∦ 00°39							
♄												
♅			☌s 04°32				□a 03°16					
♆	☌a 04°56					△a 04°52						
♇	∠s 02°11		✶a ∥ 01°50	△a 02°14								
☊				□a 00°09						⊼s 02°05		
Mc	∠s 00°39	Qa 02°06	✶s 01°00	△s 05°04		q s 00°35		✶a 03°32		☌s 02°50	∦	
Asc										□a 04°57	△a 02°52	

Chart 4a

Consultation

Feb. 20, 2001, 07:32 A.M. MST, Fountain Hills, Arizona, 111W43, 339N37

Aspect	Date	Time	Event	Type	P1 Pos.	P2 Pos	E/X/L
♅ ---- □ ☉/♃	11-02-2000	03:13 am	♅ □ ☉/♃	Ar-Na	15°♎08'	15°♑08'	Exact
♂ -- ☌ ☿	11-02-2000	10:21 am	♂ ☌ ☿	Tr-Na	29°♍07'	29°♍07'	Exact
♂ -- ∠ ♆	11-02-2000	06:45 pm	♂ ∠ ♆	Tr-Na	29°♍20'	14°♏20'	Exact
♂ -- ⚼ ♄	11-06-2000	09:53 am	♂ ⚼ ♄	Tr-Na	01°♎34'	16°♒34'℞	Exact
♆ ---- ⚼ ☉/Asc	11-10-2000	01:59 am	♆ ⚼ ☉/Asc	Ar-Na	21°♐21'	06°♌21'	Exact
♂ -- ∠ ♂	11-10-2000	05:24 am	♂ ∠ ♂	Tr-Na	03°♎54'	18°♏54'	Exact
Mc --- ☍ ☿	11-10-2000	02:18 pm	Mc ☍ ☿	Ar-Na	29°♓07'	29°♍07'	Exact
♃ -- □ ♅	11-13-2000	01:10 am	♃ □ ♅	Tr-Na	08°♊07'℞	08°♍07'	Exact
--- ☌ ♂/Asc	11-14-2000	02:54 am	☊ ☌ ♂/Asc	Ar-Na	22°♌47'	22°♌47'	Exact
♇ ---- ∠ ♀	11-14-2000	02:48 pm	♇ ∠ ♀	Tr-Na	11°♐59'	26°♎59'	Exact
♂ -- ⚼ Mc	11-15-2000	09:35 am	♂ ⚼ Mc	Tr-Na	07°♎05'	22°♒05'	Exact
☽ □ Mc	11-22-2000	12:19 pm	☽ □ Mc	Pr-Na	22°♏05'	22°♒05'	Exact
♂ -- ⚼ Asc	11-22-2000	09:59 pm	♂ ⚼ Asc	Tr-Na	11°♎40'	26°♉40'	Exact
♂ -- ☍ ♃	11-27-2000	02:37 am	♂ ☍ ♃	Tr-Na	14°♎13'	14°♈13'℞	Exact
♄ -- ☌ Asc	11-29-2000	10:45 am	♄ ☌ Asc	Tr-Na	26°♉40'℞	26°♉40'	Exact
♂ -- □ ☊	11-29-2000	03:04 pm	♂ □ ☊	Tr-Na	15°♎45'	15°♋45'℞	Exact
♂ -- ☌ ☉	11-30-2000	02:10 am	♂ ☌ ☉	Tr-Na	16°♎02'	16°♎02'	Exact
♂ -- □ ☽	12-05-2000	11:13 am	♂ □ ☽	Tr-Na	19°♎17'	19°♋17'	Exact
☿ - ⚼ ☊/Asc	12-07-2000	12:26 pm	☿ ⚼ ☊/Asc	Ar-Na	06°♏13'	21°♊13'	Exact
♂ -- ∠ ♅	12-11-2000	08:35 pm	♂ ∠ ♅	Tr-Na	23°♎07'	08°♍07'	Exact
♃ -- ∠ ☽	12-11-2000	11:15 pm	♃ ∠ ☽	Tr-Na	04°♊17'℞	19°♋17'	Exact
♇ ---- □ ♇	12-13-2000	05:19 am	♇ □ ♇	Tr-Na	13°♐05'	13°♍05'	Exact
♂ -- ☌ ♀	12-18-2000	07:32 am	♂ ☌ ♀	Tr-Na	26°♎59'	26°♎59'	Exact
♂ -- ∠ ♇	12-20-2000	03:46 am	♂ ∠ ♇	Tr-Na	28°♎05'	13°♍05'	Exact
☊ --- □ ☉	12-25-2000	07:37 am	☊ □ ☉	Tr-Na	16°♋02'℞	16°♎02'	Exact
☊ --- ☌ ☊	12-30-2000	02:41 pm	☊ ☌ ☊	Tr-Na	15°♋45'℞	15°♋45'	Exact
♅ ---- □ ♂	01-05-2001	10:59 pm	♅ □ ♂	Tr-Na	18°♒54'	18°♏54'	Exact
♂ -- ∠ ☿	01-16-2001	04:11 pm	♂ ∠ ☿	Tr-Na	14°♏07'	29°♍07'	Exact
♂ -- ☌ ♆	01-17-2001	01:17 am	♂ ☌ ♆	Tr-Na	14°♏20'	14°♏19'	Exact
♂ -- □ ♄	01-21-2001	00:04 am	♂ □ ♄	Tr-Na	16°♏34'	16°♒34'℞	Exact
Asc --- ⚼ ♂	01-24-2001	06:36 am	Asc ⚼ ♂	Ar-Na	03°♋54'	18°♏54'	Exact
♄ -- SD	01-24-2001	06:29 pm	♄ SD	Tr-Na	24°♉04'		
♃ -- SD	01-25-2001	03:13 am	♃ SD	Tr-Na	01°♊11'		
♂ -- ☌ ♂	01-25-2001	04:18 am	♂ ☌ ♂	Tr-Na	18°♏54'	18°♏54'	Exact
☿ - □ ☉/Asc	01-27-2001	07:23 am	☿ □ ☉/Asc	Ar-Na	06°♏21'	06°♌21'	Exact
Mc --- ⚼ ♆	01-27-2001	07:43 pm	Mc ⚼ ♆	Ar-Na	29°♓20'	14°♏20'	Exact
☊ --- □ ♃	01-28-2001	11:22 am	☊ □ ♃	Tr-Na	14°♋13'℞	14°♈13'℞	Exact
♂ -- □ Mc	01-30-2001	09:41 pm	♂ □ Mc	Tr-Na	22°♏05'	22°♒05'	Exact
♂ -- ☍ ♃/♅	02-04-2001	01:16 pm	♂ ☍ ♃/♅	Ar-Na	26°♐10'	26°♊10'	Exact
♂ -- ☍ Asc	02-08-2001	08:32 am	♂ ☍ Asc	Tr-Na	26°♏40'	26°♉40'	Exact
♂ -- ⚼ ♃	02-13-2001	03:38 am	♂ ⚼ ♃	Tr-Na	29°♏13'	14°♈13'℞	Exact
♂ -- ⚼ ☊	02-16-2001	01:35 am	♂ ⚼ ☊	Tr-Na	00°♐45'	15°♋45'℞	Exact
♂ -- ∠ ☉	02-16-2001	02:30 pm	♂ ∠ ☉	Tr-Na	01°♐02'	16°♎02'	Exact
♀ - ⚼ ☽	02-17-2001	11:07 am	♀ ⚼ ☽	Ar-Na	04°♐17'	19°♋17'	Exact
♂ -- ⚼ ☽	02-22-2001	10:32 pm	♂ ⚼ ☽	Tr-Na	04°♐17'	19°♋17'	Exact
--- ⚼ ♇/☊	02-28-2001	10:40 pm	Mc ⚼ ♇/☊	Ar-Na	29°♓25'	14°♌25'	Exact
♂ -- □ ♅	03-02-2001	04:43 pm	♂ □ ♅	Tr-Na	08°♐07'	08°♍07'	Exact
♅ ---- ☌ Mc	03-03-2001	10:52 am	♅ ☌ Mc	Tr-Na	22°♒05'	22°♒05'	Exact
♃ -- ∠ ☽	03-10-2001	05:43 am	♃ ∠ ☽	Tr-Na	04°♊17'	19°♋17'	Exact
♂ -- ∠ ♀	03-10-2001	08:56 pm	♂ ∠ ♀	Tr-Na	11°♐59'	26°♎59'	Exact
♂ -- □ ♇	03-13-2001	06:49 am	♂ □ ♇	Tr-Na	13°♐05'	13°♍05'	Exact
☊ --- ∠ Asc	03-17-2001	03:26 pm	☊ ∠ Asc	Tr-Na	11°♋40'℞	26°♉40'	Exact
♇ ---- SR℞	03-17-2001	04:24 pm	♇ SR℞	Tr-Na	15°♐17'℞		
♄ -- ☌ Asc	03-20-2001	06:03 am	♄ ☌ Asc	Tr-Na	26°♉40'	26°♉40'	Exact
☽ □ Asc	03-21-2001	11:24 pm	☽ □ Asc	Ar-Na	26°♌40'	26°♉40'	Exact
♃ -- ∠ ♄/Asc	03-23-2001	03:36 am	♃ ∠ ♄/Asc	Ar-Na	21°♉37'	06°♈37'	Exact
♃ -- □ ♅	04-03-2001	03:42 pm	♃ □ ♅	Tr-Na	08°♊07'	08°♍07'	Exact
♃ -- ∠ ☿/♃	04-09-2001	06:34 pm	♃ ∠ ☿/♃	Ar-Na	21°♉40'	06°♋40'	Exact
♆ ---- ☌ ♀/♄	04-10-2001	10:18 pm	♆ ☌ ♀/♄	Ar-Na	21°♐46'	21°♐46'	Exact
☽ ☍ Asc	04-13-2001	06:27 am	☽ ☍ Asc	Pr-Na	26°♏40'	26°♉40'	Exact
♄ -- ∠ ♃	04-14-2001	00:58 am	♄ ∠ ♃	Tr-Na	29°♉13'	14°♈13'℞	Exact
--- ☍ ☉/♇	04-20-2001	05:30 pm	Mc ☍ ☉/♇	Ar-Na	29°♓33'	29°♍33'	Exact

M=☿ 2,5

♂♄☌A, 2nd time

→ filed for divorce

♂☊□☊7, 1st time

♂♅☌M, 1st

♂♄☌A, final

→ to subpoena "other woman"

SP☽☌VII

striving for power and control

"Julia" Time Flow

Aspect	Date	Time	Event	Type	P1 Pos.	P2 Pos	E/X/L
♃ -- ⚼ ♀	04-23-2001	01:47 pm	♃ ⚼ ♀	Tr-Na	11°♊59'	26°♎59'	Exact
♄ -- ∠ ☊	04-26-2001	10:24 pm	♄ ∠ ☊	Tr-Na	00°♊45'	15°♋45'℞	Exact
♃ -- □ ♇	04-28-2001	07:59 pm	♃ □ ♇	Tr-Na	13°♊05'	13°♍05'	Exact
♄ -- ⚼ ☉	04-29-2001	05:09 am	♄ ⚼ ☉	Tr-Na	01°♊02'	16°♎02'	Exact
♇ ---- □ ♀/♃	05-09-2001	04:21 pm	♇ □ ♀/♃	Ar-Na	20°♎36'	20°♑36'	Exact
♆ ---- SR	05-10-2001	02:56 pm	♆ SR	Tr-Na	08°♒47'℞		
♂ -- SR	05-11-2001	10:43 am	♂ SR	Tr-Na	29°♐03'℞		
♄ -- ∠ ☽	05-24-2001	04:49 pm	♄ ∠ ☽	Tr-Na	04°♊17'	19°♋17'	Exact
♅ ---- SR	05-29-2001	07:40 am	♅ SR	Tr-Na	24°♒50'℞		
☊ --- ⚼ Mc	06-12-2001	08:32 am	☊ ⚼ Mc	Tr-Na	07°♋05'℞	22°♒05'	Exact
♅ ---- □ ☊	06-16-2001	04:42 am	♅ □ ☊	Ar-Na	15°♎45'	15°♋45'℞	Exact
--- ⚼ ♄/Mc	06-23-2001	11:22 am	Asc ⚼ ♄/Mc	Ar-Na	04°♋19'	19°♒19'	Exact
♄ -- □ ♅	06-23-2001	10:20 pm	♄ □ ♅	Tr-Na	08°♊07'	08°♍07'	Exact
☿ - ∠ ♀/♄	06-28-2001	03:21 am	☿ ∠ ♀/♄	Ar-Na	06°♏46'	21°♐46'	Exact
♇ ---- □ ♇	07-07-2001	10:43 pm	♇ □ ♇	Tr-Na	13°♐05'℞	13°♍05'	Exact
♃ -- □ ☿	07-08-2001	07:15 pm	♃ □ ☿	Tr-Na	29°♊07'	29°♍07'	Exact
♃ -- ⚼ ♆	07-09-2001	06:22 pm	♃ ⚼ ♆	Tr-Na	29°♊20'	14°♏20'	Exact
♂ -- SD	07-19-2001	05:44 pm	♂ SD	Tr-Na	15°♐07'		
♃ -- ⚼ ♄	07-19-2001	09:27 pm	♃ ⚼ ♄	Tr-Na	01°♋34'	16°♒34'℞	Exact
♄ -- ⚼ ♀	07-29-2001	05:35 am	♄ ⚼ ♀	Tr-Na	11°♊59'	26°♎59'	Exact
♃ -- ⚼ ♂	07-30-2001	09:14 pm	♃ ⚼ ♂	Tr-Na	03°♋54'	18°♏54'	Exact
♅ ---- ∠ ☉/☊	08-05-2001	11:22 pm	♅ ∠ ☉/☊	Ar-Na	15°♎54'	00°♍54'	Exact
♄ -- □ ♇	08-11-2001	02:00 am	♄ □ ♇	Tr-Na	13°♊05'	13°♍05'	Exact
☊ --- ⚼ ♂	08-11-2001	06:54 am	☊ ⚼ ♂	Tr-Na	03°♋54'℞	18°♏54'	Exact
♃ -- ⚼ Mc	08-15-2001	06:08 pm	♃ ⚼ Mc	Tr-Na	07°♋05'	22°♒05'	Exact
♇ ---- SD	08-23-2001	06:41 am	♇ SD	Tr-Na	12°♐32'		
♅ ---- ☌ Mc	09-04-2001	11:30 am	♅ ☌ Mc	Tr-Na	22°♒05'℞	22°♒05'	Exact
♂ -- □ ☿	09-06-2001	06:27 pm	♂ □ ☿	Tr-Na	29°♐07'	29°♍07'	Exact
♃ -- □ Mc	09-06-2001	10:10 pm	♃ □ Mc	Ar-Na	22°♉05'	22°♒05'	Exact
♂ -- ∠ ♆	09-07-2001	04:48 am	♂ ∠ ♆	Tr-Na	29°♐20'	14°♏20'	Exact
♅ ---- ☌ ♂/♇	09-11-2001	03:02 am	♅ ☌ ♂/♇	Ar-Na	15°♎59'	15°♎59'	Exact
♂ -- ∠ ♄	09-11-2001	01:14 pm	♂ ∠ ♄	Tr-Na	01°♑34'	16°♒34'℞	Exact
♃ -- ∠ Asc	09-11-2001	09:23 pm	♃ ∠ Asc	Tr-Na	11°♋40'	26°♉40'	Exact
♂ -- ∠ ♂	09-15-2001	09:49 pm	♂ ∠ ♂	Tr-Na	03°♑54'	18°♏54'	Exact
♀ - ⚼ ♇/Asc	09-20-2001	05:35 am	♀ ⚼ ♇/Asc	Ar-Na	04°♐52'	19°♋52'	Exact
♂ -- ∠ Mc	09-21-2001	01:04 pm	♂ ∠ Mc	Tr-Na	07°♑05'	22°♒05'	Exact
☊ --- ⚼ ♄	09-24-2001	01:27 pm	☊ ⚼ ♄	Tr-Na	01°♋34'℞	16°♒34'℞	Exact
♅ ---- ☌ ☉	09-25-2001	05:58 pm	♅ ☌ ☉	Ar-Na	16°♎02'	16°♎02'	Exact
♄ -- SR	09-26-2001	06:30 pm	♄ SR	Tr-Na	14°♊58'℞		
♂ -- ⚼ ♀/Asc	09-29-2001	05:52 am	♂ ⚼ ♀/Asc	Ar-Na	26°♐50'	11°♌50'	Exact
♂ -- ⚼ Asc	09-29-2001	07:08 am	♂ ⚼ Asc	Tr-Na	11°♑40'	26°♉40'	Exact
♃ -- □ ♃	10-03-2001	02:34 am	♃ □ ♃	Tr-Na	14°♋13'	14°♈13'℞	Exact
♂ -- □ ♃	10-03-2001	10:44 am	♂ □ ♃	Tr-Na	14°♑13'	14°♈13'℞	Exact
♂ -- ☍ ☊	10-05-2001	09:22 pm	♂ ☍ ☊	Tr-Na	15°♑45'	15°♋45'℞	Exact
♂ -- □ ☉	10-06-2001	08:03 am	♂ □ ☉	Tr-Na	16°♑02'	16°♎02'	Exact
♇ ---- □ ♇	10-07-2001	03:02 am	♇ □ ♇	Tr-Na	13°♐05'	13°♍05'	Exact

Business Plans

meetings

♄□♇, 2nd

♄ ♅☌M, 2nd

danger of attack

♅=☉ ★

END

♄□♇, final

"Julia" Time Flow (Cont'd)

the consultation. The most powerful measurement symbology occurs in September 2001 with SA Uranus=Sun. Working backwards from this peak, we can determine the stepping-stones of development toward it. Note as well that the outer planets almost always make transit aspects to planets and Angles *three times* (direct, retrograde, direct), and that this observation is sometimes very important in analytical consideration, favoring the "final hit."

When Julia told me that she was planning to divorce her husband, I asked her (the consultation taking place February 20, 2001) immediately what had occurred *in relation to this decision* in very late November, early December 2000. Julia said she filed for divorce on December 5. Note tr Mars conjunct her Sun and square her Moon at the "same time" as tr Saturn was conjoined with her Ascendant and the SP Moon was square her Midheaven. A peak time indeed, with the Mars transit as trigger within the period. Additionally, note tr Pluto square Pluto, ruler of her 7th, a transit that always connotes "a new way, a new perspective" involving the House Pluto rules or in which it is placed or both.

I suggested that there could be another major development in early March, about ten days after the consultation (the measurements centered on tr Uranus conjunct the MC (the first contact) and the *final* touch of tr Saturn upon the Ascendant, with the important angular measurement *SP Moon square the Ascendant*). Julia said that, at that time, her lawyer was going to introduce the subpoena of "the other woman" involved.

I then suggested that this would spark things strongly, with her making a power move shortly thereafter in mid-April, with SP Moon conjunct the Descendant and SA MC=Sun/Pluto, with Pluto ruling her 7th: "Striving for power and control; power games with important consequences." At the same time, with Pluto=Venus/Jupiter, a picture of much enthusiasm and popularity, Julia said that there were some important business considerations possible at that time. I suggested that we talk about that developmental theme separately a bit later in our discussion.

I advised her that there could be a very strong counterattack from her husband early in September (Uranus=Mars-Pluto). I asked about the possibility of *physical* attack by her husband; she said that her husband had never hit her, and I countered that this would then undoubtedly be a legal move, a court move, that despite its aggressive nature would probably lead to the end—settlement two weeks later, decidedly to her benefit: Uranus=Sun with tr Jupiter square Jupiter and the final transiting square of Pluto to its natal position, Pluto ruling her 7th.

Our conversation was rich with detailed strategies, careful value judgments, and objectivity.

Then, I switched tracks with Julia, still following the pronounced Uranian theme of the measurements, with Uranus ruling her Midheaven: I asked her if she were thinking of changing jobs or starting her own business. Julia answered the question with a resounding "Yes!" and proceeded to talk about all the considerations.

The same measurements outlining the reality of her divorce proceedings were used to accentuate her individual professional development away from her present job and into business for herself with the SA Uranus=Sun measurement partile in September 2001, extending into December as a backdrop for tr Uranus making its final conjunction contact with her Midheaven (not shown here).

Julia had sensed/discovered her husband's affair two years into their marriage. She again questioned her ability to make the right choices for relationship. Here her second marriage was quickly in trouble. She said that she was "repeating her pattern."

Natally, Pluto, her 7th House significator, is highly charged by the Uranus square, and her Venus is peregrine, dissociated from relationship security, yearning for it. We see her Saturn$_{Rx}$; the evidence of a highly important mother figure, taking care of things (Sun square the Nodal Axis); her Ptolemeicly unaspected Mercury in Virgo, ruling the 5th, quindecile Jupiter ruling the 8th (the mind extremely caught up with sexual intent, now suffering frustration and humiliation yet again); and the background models for marriage established in the culture of the South American country in which she was born.

Julia was repeating a pattern indeed, as so many of us do, a pattern to which she is vividly vulnerable.

Chart 26: "Toni"

A Protectionistic/Defeating Bubble: Toni's horoscope (p. 160) shows a classic, clear father attachment (a longing for what was not provided): Saturn$_{Rx}$ is

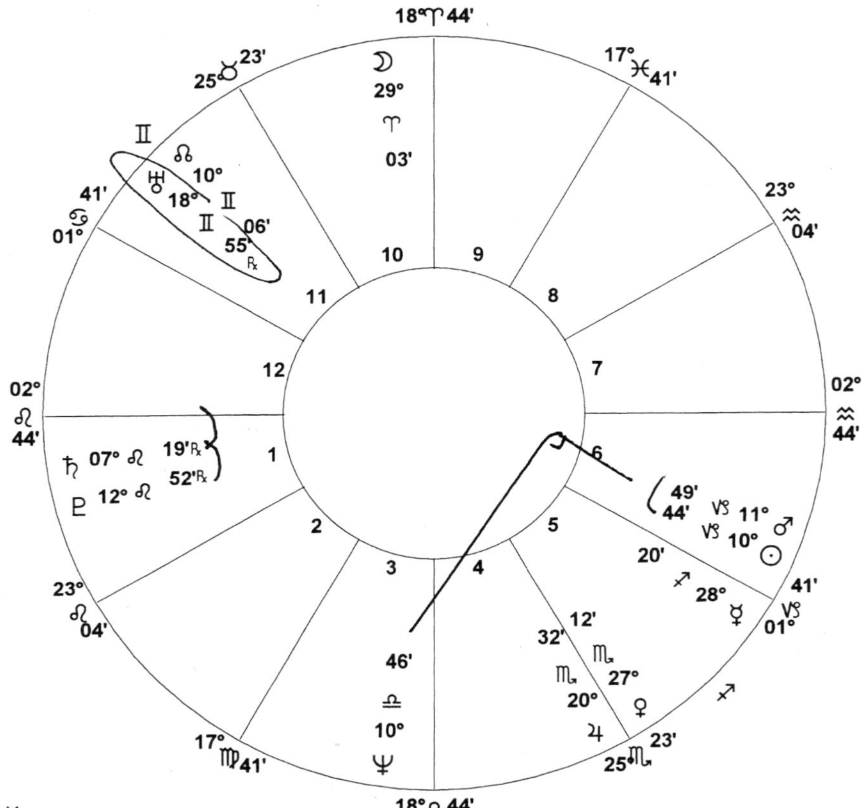

	☽	☉	☿	♀	♂	♃	♄	♅	♆	♇	☊	Mc
☉												
☿	△s 00°43	∥										
♀	⊼s 01°51	∠a 01°29										
♂		☌a∥ 01°05	∥	∠a 00°23								
♃				☌s 06°40								
♄												
♅		⋕	⋕		⋕	⊼s 01°37						
♆		□a 00°03		∠s 01°26	□s 01°02		✶s 03°27					
♇		⊼a⋕ 02°09	Qs⋕ 00°27		⊼a⋕ 01°04		☌s 05°33	∥	✶a 02°06			
☊		⊼s 00°38			⊼s 01°43		✶s 02°47		△s 00°41	✶s 02°46		
Mc	∥					⊼a 01°48		✶a 00°11		△s 05°52		
Asc	□s 03°41			△s 05°32			☌a∥ 04°35	∠a 01°11				

Chart 26

"Toni"

conjoined with Pluto and is also conjoined the Ascendant, i.e., at the heart of her being. It intrudes on her nascent "queen complex."

This beginning of her portrait is extended dramatically through the peregrine Uranus—a touch of eccentricism here, independence, in the light of the Leo Ascendant and the Aries Moon. She comes first, is *numero uno*. What did the father think? How did he support this? What was deficient here?

"My father died when I was seven years old [SA Asc=Saturn/Pluto ("Sadness, mourning") with tr Saturn square Saturn-Pluto, September-November 1954] and, from that overwhelming incident, I created a paradigm that was repeated often. [While] my father was a hard-working man who did support his family when he was alive, I did not focus on that though. When he died, there was not enough insurance and my mother had to work several jobs just to try and make ends meet. I worked very hard in school to improve myself **so I would never have to depend on a man.**"

The dissociation (peregrination) of Uranus, ruler of the 7th is astounding corroborative of Patti's reality experience: there is a desperate need here to relate, but a bubble warning that it will never be reliable.

"I did not have a break-through with my problem until about a year ago (she is fifty-three). I caught myself telling someone that 'You can never depend on a man.' And what do you think I had attracted in the past: weak men who can not support themselves." [Her time of understanding, finally.]

Patti has finally found someone persuasively strong and is off-the-wall enthusiastic about the relationship.

Chart 27: "Elizabeth"

When discussing relationship break-up, divorce, when we ask ourselves *when did the break-up begin*, we understand easily that it begins even *before* the relationship (marriage) starts: the tug-of-life between societal prescriptions and individual needs, toeing the mark to gain acceptance, victimization by the modeling of marriage by our parents, participation with the idealized projections expected of us, creating bubbles begging to burst—*all this takes place before the relationship does*. Here is yet another clear-cut case that focused all the accumulated developmental tension on the very day of the marriage ceremony!

"Elizabeth's" horoscope (p. 163) suggests that she gives herself away to others (Western Hemisphere emphasis), but stays deeply private to herself defensively. Her identity is extremely cerebral (the Gemini focus, Mercury prominence on an Angle, augmented by the square from Jupiter; the Moon in Sagittarius, the Pluto power conjunction with Mars, ruler of the mindset 3rd; AP=Mercury/Pluto). At the same time, the cerebration takes on definite dimensions of vulnerability: Neptune=Mercury/Pluto ("overdoing the mental issues to the point of draining energies") and Saturn=Mercury/Asc ("adopting a strategic reserve in expression, *withdrawal from the social circle*, protecting the position").

So what might be behind this posture? The horoscope is dominated by Saturn opposed the Moon. Indeed, the orb is wide, but the opposition *must* be valid: we see the powerful Mars-Pluto conjunction, with Pluto ruling one arm of the parental axis, and Saturn opposition with the Moon would fit the parental tension analysis perfectly.

Additionally the Uranus-Venus conjunction is *quindecile to the Midheaven*, Uranus ruling the Ascendant and Venus ruling the parental 4th holding the conjunction. This suggests very strongly that Elizabeth will define her identity insistently through the work she does (she is a very skilled astrologer); evaluation of her work takes the place of evaluation of who she really is, a clearly defensive life organization. As well, the quindecile here shows enormous, intense tension with one of the parents, or both in this case, affecting her personal development strongly.

Her self-worth profile is jeopardized also (Neptune$_2$ square Saturn$_{12}$), and the battleground from these early home tensions will probably manifest in relationships (Mars-Pluto-Node conjunct the Descendant, opposing the Ascendant; Uranus, through its conjunction with Venus is brought into conjunction with the Sun, ruler of the 7th).

Here, Elizabeth speaks about her horoscope:

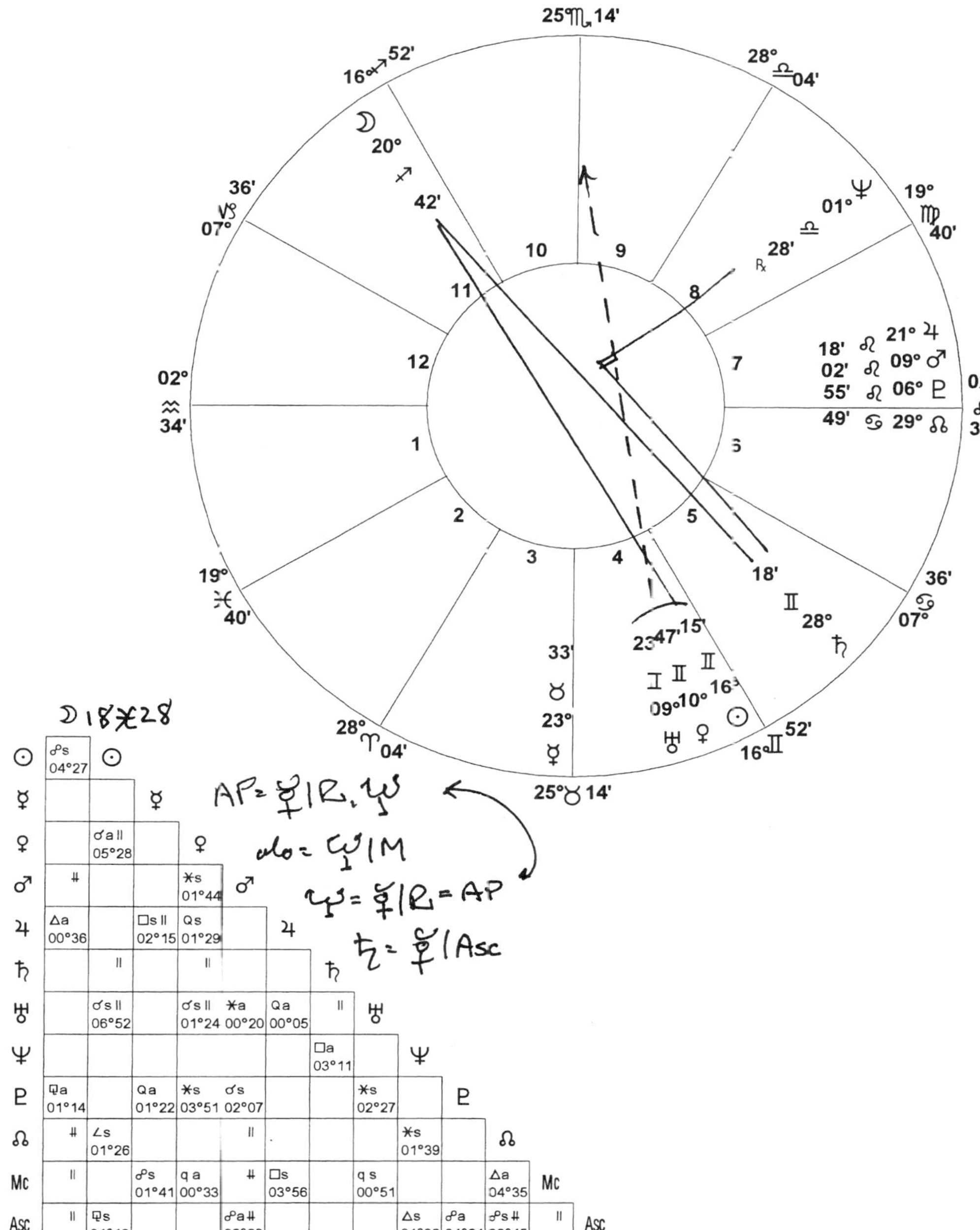

Chart 27

"Elizabeth"

> The difficulty in relationships was integrated into my perspective with my dependency for survival upon my father (after my mother's death when I was age nine) with whom I could not allow myself to become emotionally close because of my fear of him (he was a functional alcoholic with a violent temper). My view of the world was, *"I was safe as long as I did not become too close to the person who I depended upon to be safe."*

This is a vivid statement of the Western Hemisphere emphasis and the simultaneous withdrawal tendencies.

> Saturn in the 5th suggests my resistance to opening up my heart fully to give love . . . for fear of being hurt. Saturn opposed the Moon suggests my difficulty to receive the emotional nurturing that I longed for as a child. The Sun opposed Moon suggests the diametrically opposed positions of my parents and their disturbance at my being born.
>
> Mother would kick my little bed and growl, "I wish you had never been born!" I would be playing with my dolls as if they were babies, and my mother was say, "Women are stupid to have babies." Then, after mother died, an aunt told me that my mother and father had tried to abort me [a doctor's effort failed].
>
> I learned as well from my aunt that my grandmother had tried to abort my mother!
>
> The rippling aftermath of my feelings of being unwanted carries over into an adulthood of feeling fear of intimate relationships. All of this operated on an unconscious level when I was younger, but now it is all very apparent to me.
>
> Saturn square Neptune suggests my illusions of how love relationships "work" based on my behavioral pattern to "give myself (power) away" in relationships (along with the Western Hemisphere emphasis).
>
> I see now that it was no coincidence that I married a man who declared to me as we walked to the justice of the peace on our wedding day that "we will just get divorced if we don't like being married,

> right?" that I attracted a man who specifically desired to live alone, who clearly did not want children to complicate his freedom, and that I lived alone for fourteen years after my marriage dissolved.

In my own relationship life (Noel Tyl, p. 36), my first marriage broke up with SA Pluto =MC and tr Mars-Saturn conjunct my Ascendant, Saturn ruling the 7th. A long-term relationship thereafter dissolved with tr Pluto on the lady's Ascendant; an important relationship thereafter dissolved with tr Saturn, ruling the 7th, conjoining my Sun in the 7th. My present marriage is currently threatened (2000–2001) with SA Uranus=Sun in the 7th, with "final test" transits coming in mid-2002, when tr Saturn squares natal Saturn as tr Pluto squares it also.

Charts 28, 29: "Ian" and "Corinne"

"Ian" came to me with quite a love-sick request: "Was there anything I could do to tell him if this lady he desired so would go off with him on quite a spectacular and long trip; could their relationship happen?" Ian made an appointment for himself and separately for the lady, "Corinne."

Ian's horoscope (p. 166) clearly is dominated by Saturn square the horizon upon which the Moon is in exact conjunction. The Uranus square with Mercury$_{Rx}$ brings in the anxiety of being unlovable (Mercury ruling the 11th). AP=Saturn/Neptune clearly suggests a sad-sack, depressed demeanor. Node= Moon/Pluto suggests grand emotionalism; probably meeting up with headstrong women who easily take advantage of him (Saturn square with the Moon powerfully located in the 7th; Mercury ruling the 7th squared by Uranus) in an out-and-out power struggle (Pluto=Sun/Moon). Idealism about relationship is always at hand and in mind: Mercury$_{7, 11}$ sextile Venus.

Ian is very wealthy: Jupiter square the Sun$_M$-Nodal axis (and here it was important to study Ian's maternal relationship in connection with his model for his female relationships).

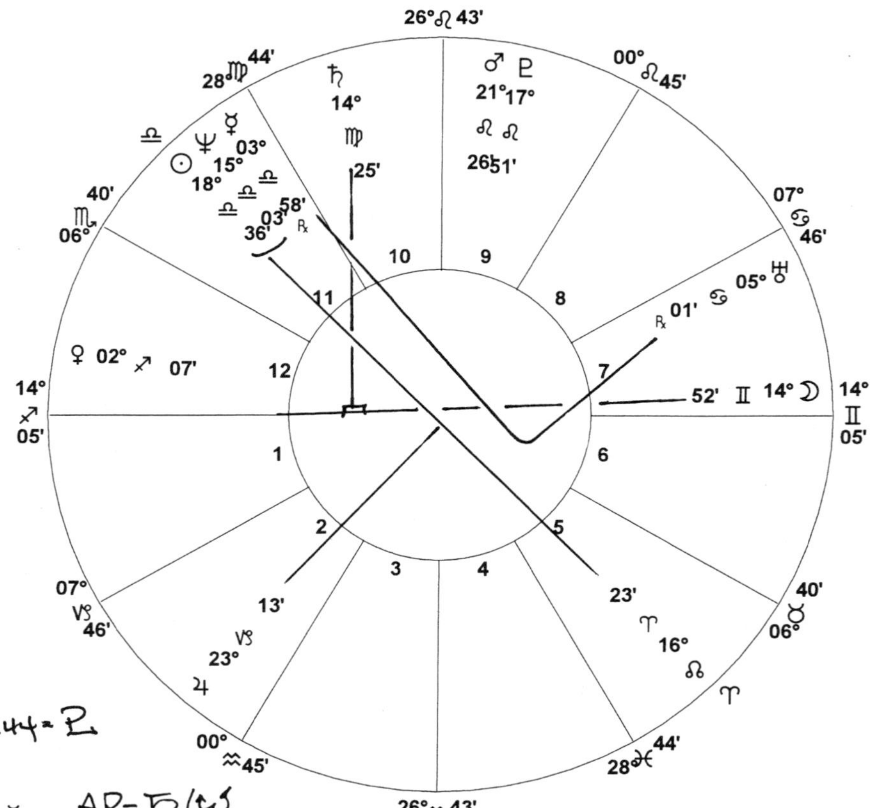

☽ 16♈44 = ♇

AP = ♄/♆

alo = ☽/♇

♇ = ☉/☽

♀ = ♂/♄

	☽	☉	☿	♀	♂	♃	♄	♅	♆	♇	☊	Mc
☉	△a 03°44											
☿												
♀		∠a 01°29	✶a 01°51									
♂		✶a 02°51	∠s 02°28									
♃		□a 04°37		∥	⊼a 01°47							
♄	□s 00°27	#										
♅			□s 01°03	#	∠s 01°25							
♆	△a 00°11	☌s 03°33		∠s 02°04								
♇	✶a 02°59	✶s 00°44	∠a 01°07	#	☌s 03°35	#		∠a ∥ 02°10	✶a 02°48			
☊	✶a 01°31	☍s # 02°13		⚻s 00°44	△s 05°03		⊼a 01°59		☍a 01°20	△s 01°28		
Mc	Qa 00°09			□a 05°24	☌s 05°16							
Asc	☍a 00°48		Qa 01°54	∥		∥	□a 00°20		✶a 00°59	△a # 03°47	△a 02°19	

Chart 28

"Ian"

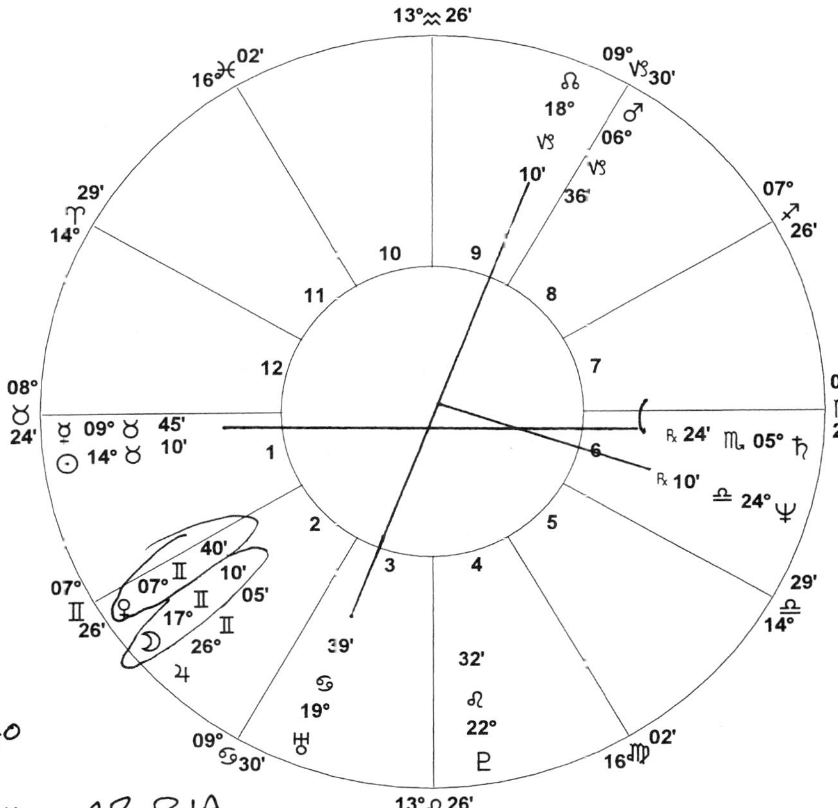

☽ 0♊40

AP = ♇/A
♄♆ = ♃/♇
♄ = ♇/☊
♇ = ♀/♄

	☽	☉	☿	♀	♂	♃	♄	♅	♆	♇	☊	Mc
☉												
☿		☌a 04°25										
♀												
♂	#		△s 03°09	⊼s 01°04								
♃			∠a 01°20	∥								
♄			☍s 04°21	⊼s 02°16	⚹s 01°12							
♅			Qs 02°06	∥	q s 01°57	∥						
♆			q s 00°35	⚼a 01°29	Qs 00°26	△s 01°55		□a 04°31				
♇					⚼a 00°56	⚹s ∥ 03°33	Qa 00°52	∥	⚹a 01°38			
☊	⊼a 01°01	△a 04°00		#			Qs 00°46	☍s # 01°29	□s 06°00			
Mc	△a 03°44	□a # 00°44	□s 03°41	△s 05°46		⚼s 02°21						
Asc		☌a 05°46	☌a ∥ 01°21		△s 01°48		☍s 03°00	Qs 00°45	q a 00°46			□s 05°02

Chart 29

"Corinne"

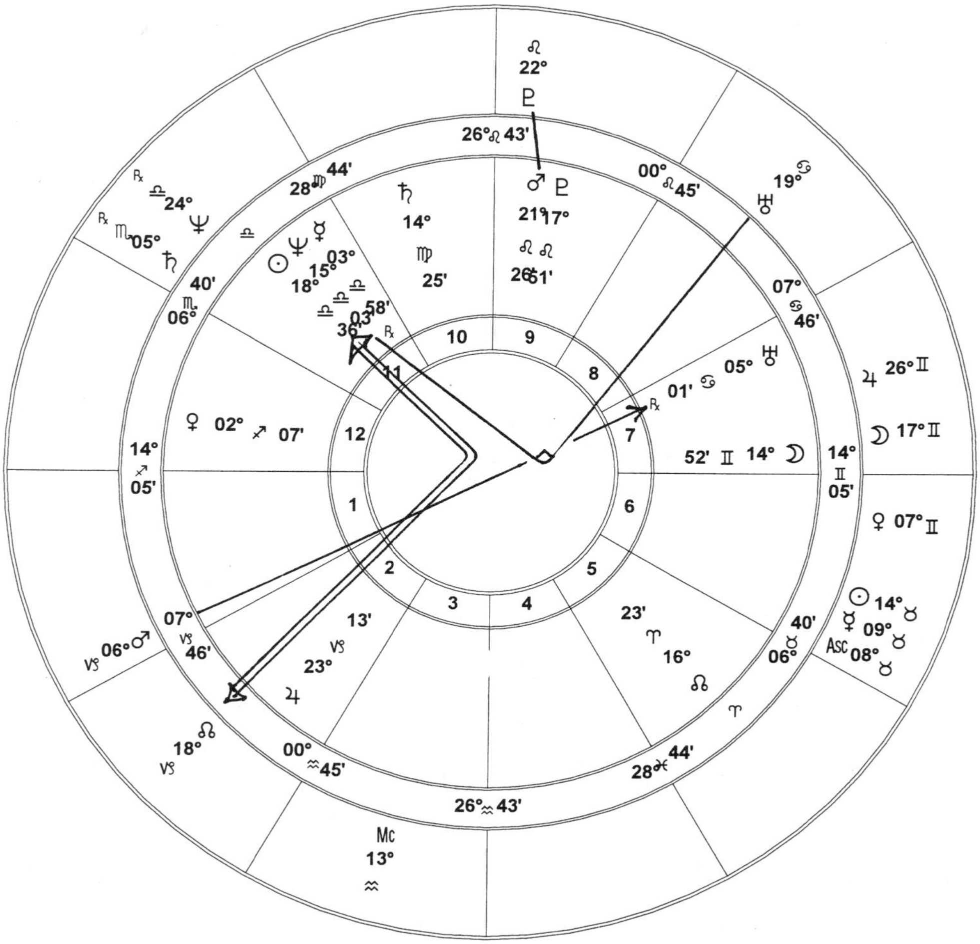

Chart 30

Inner Chart
"Ian"

Outer Chart
"Corinne"

Corinne's horoscope (p. 167) has the Saturn$_{Rx}$ phenomenon on her seventh cusp, with a fractured self-worth profile with Mercury quindecile Neptune, ruler of the 11th! Uranus, one of her parental rulers, is conjunct the Nodal axis and quindecile Mars. The classic pattern of early home difficulties is shown here, as we have seen it in so many different but related ways in cases supporting this book.

The Moon is peregrine in Gemini: the reigning motivator of Corrine's life will be to get tied in, to get connected, associated somehow through relationships, and the many different ways to do that will be entertained by her mind.

Venus, ruler of her Ascendant, is peregrine as well! Corinne desperately needs connections to others to know who she is and to get where she wants to go.

Two midpoint pictures that are especially apt to complete Corinne's portrait: Neptune=Jupiter/Pluto, "the inclination to be deceptive, working a situation into one's own format"; Pluto=Venus/Saturn, "unusually strong tensions toward separation."

It was clear that Ian desired Corinne, and that Corinne was considering exploiting him. He wanted to take her under his wing and tour grandly with her to set her up in her art career. She found that most attractive, but relationships are very difficult for Corinne.

Chart 30 (p. 168) shows Ian and Corinne together in double-ringed format. Note the contacts:

- Corinne's Uranus squares Ian's Sun
- Her Mars opposes his Uranus
- Her Pluto conjoins his Mars.

These are extremely powerful, attacking measurements; a power struggle in the offing, for sure.

- And finally—unexpected indeed—Corrine's *Nodal Axis is exactly square Ian's Sun.* This is the powerful attraction Ian feels for her.

Ian kept repeating to me that he wanted to "help her." In the light of the Nodal contact with his Sun, I allowed myself to entertain the thought that maybe, just maybe there was some kind of debt here from some other time, that Ian had to repay Corinne, *and she felt it.* In a rare editorialization within the consultation process, I urged them to go on the trip together: Ian had to give it a shot, if only to rid his life system of the pressure; Corrine's rewards were obvious.

The time-flow charts that follow (pp. 171–174) tell the story, especially dramatically from Corinne's perspective and her astrology.

She had lost her job at the end of 1999 with the Uranus final transit of her Midheaven as tr Saturn conjoined her Sun (October 31) and square her Midheaven. But then look at the reward time in April-May 2000 with tr Jupiter square her Midheaven, then conjoining her Sun, with SP Moon at the MC as well! This is tremendous change of status (I noted that her Jupiter ruled the 8th, other's resources).

Ian's time-flow chart in the same time period (pp. 175–176) shows MC= Sun/Node, success through associations and tr Saturn square the Midheaven, all working on the backdrop of Jupiter=Ascendant, enthusiasm and harmony, possible travel, and Venus=Jupiter, happiness in love, success, etc. During the trip they split in argument and then got back together to complete the tour. The relationship ended in January 2001 tr Pluto conjunct Ian's Ascendant-Descendant axis, squaring his Saturn, and opposing his Moon.

The end for Corinne was corroborated by Sun=Saturn/Pluto, "enforced change separation," the build-up of her accumulated semisquare solar Arc in March 2001 with tr Uranus opposed Pluto, ruler of her 7th.

The reason for Corinne's clash with Ian was certainly a burst bubble, a bubble that was probably ultrafragile to begin with; there is a thin line between love and money (viewed through the 2nd House profile), and her motives were clearly orientated to career advancement in the light of her major life changes. Her projections upon Ian were temporary and strategically cramped. Ian's projections upon Corrine were equally as fragile, built upon lost job

Aspect	Date	Time	Event	Type	P1 Pos.	P2 Pos	E/X/L
♂ -- ∠ ☊	09-07-1999	02:53 pm	♂ ∠ ☊	Tr-Na	03°♐10'	18°♑10'℞	Exact
☊ — ∠ ♃	09-09-1999	07:27 am	☊ ∠ ♃	Tr-Na	11°♌05'℞	26°♊05'	Exact
♂ -- ⚻ ♅	09-09-1999	10:06 pm	♂ ⚻ ♅	Tr-Na	04°♐39'	19°♋39'	Exact
♂ -- ☍ ♀	09-14-1999	01:38 pm	♂ ☍ ♀	Tr-Na	07°♐40'	07°♊40'	Exact
♅ — ☌ Mc	09-14-1999	10:47 pm	♅ ☌ Mc	Tr-Na	13°♒26'℞	13°♒26'	Exact
♂ -- ∠ ♆	09-16-1999	07:52 pm	♂ ∠ ♆	Tr-Na	09°♐10'	24°♎10'℞	Exact
♂ -- ☍ ☽	09-28-1999	03:46 pm	♂ ☍ ☽	Tr-Na	17°♐10'	17°♊10'	Exact
☿ - □ ♆/♇	09-30-1999	04:33 am	☿ □ ♆/♇	Ar-Na	23°♊21'	23°♍21'	Exact
♂ -- ∠ ♄	10-03-1999	08:12 am	♂ ∠ ♄	Tr-Na	20°♐24'	05°♏24'℞	Exact
☊ — □ ☿	10-04-1999	10:23 am	☊ □ ☿	Tr-Na	09°♌45'℞	09°♉45'	Exact
♃ -- ∠ ☽	10-06-1999	11:59 am	♃ ∠ ☽	Tr-Na	02°♉10'℞	17°♊10'	Exact
♂ -- ⚻ Asc	10-07-1999	02:44 pm	♂ ⚻ Asc	Tr-Na	23°♐24'	08°♉24'	Exact
♂ -- ⚻ ☿	10-09-1999	12:23 pm	♂ ⚻ ☿	Tr-Na	24°♐45'	09°♉45'	Exact
♂ -- ☍ ♃	10-11-1999	09:19 am	♂ ☍ ♃	Tr-Na	26°♐05'	26°♊05'	Exact
♆ — SD	10-13-1999	04:34 pm	♆ SD	Tr-Na	01°♒35'		
♂ -- ∠ Mc	10-14-1999	04:22 pm	♂ ∠ Mc	Tr-Na	28°♐26'	13°♒26'	Exact
♂ -- ⚻ ☉	10-15-1999	04:50 pm	♂ ⚻ ☉	Tr-Na	29°♐10'	14°♉10'	Exact
☽ ☍ ☊/Mc	10-16-1999	02:42 am	☽ ☍ ☊/Mc	Ar-Na	00°♌48'	00°♒48'	Exact
☿ - ∠ Asc	10-21-1999	00:43 am	☿ ∠ Asc	Ar-Na	23°♊24'	08°♉24'	Exact
♅ — SD	10-22-1999	09:24 pm	♅ SD	Tr-Na	12°♒52'		
☽ □ ♄	10-24-1999	07:04 pm	☽ □ ♄	Pr-Na	05°♒24'	05°♏24'℞	Exact
♂ -- ☌ ♂	10-25-1999	10:20 pm	♂ ☌ ♂	Tr-Na	06°♑36'	06°♑36'	Exact
♃ -- □ ☿	10-26-1999	02:38 pm	♃ □ ☿	Ar-Na	09°♌45'	09°♉45'	Exact
♂ -- ⚻ ♇	10-27-1999	04:46 am	♂ ⚻ ♇	Tr-Na	07°♑32'	22°♌32'	Exact
☊ — □ Asc	10-29-1999	07:55 pm	☊ □ Asc	Tr-Na	08°♌24'℞	08°♉24'	Exact
♄ -- ☌ ☉	10-31-1999	01:47 pm	♄ ☌ ☉	Tr-Na	14°♉10'℞	14°♉10'	Exact
♇ — ∠ ♆	11-01-1999	11:29 am	♇ ∠ ♆	Tr-Na	09°♐10'	24°♎10'℞	Exact
♄ -- □ Mc	11-09-1999	03:44 pm	♄ □ Mc	Tr-Na	13°♉26'℞	13°♒26'	Exact
♃ -- ☌ ☉/♄	11-10-1999	02:34 am	♃ ☌ ☉/♄	Ar-Na	09°♌47'	09°♌47'	Exact
♂ -- ☌ ☊	11-10-1999	11:48 am	♂ ☌ ☊	Tr-Na	18°♑10'	18°♑10'℞	Exact
♂ -- ☍ ♅	11-12-1999	10:52 am	♂ ☍ ♅	Tr-Na	19°♑39'	19°♋39'	Exact
♂ -- ⚻ ♀	11-16-1999	10:58 am	♂ ⚻ ♀	Tr-Na	22°♑40'	07°♊40'	Exact
♂ -- □ ♆	11-18-1999	10:09 am	♂ □ ♆	Tr-Na	24°♑10'	24°♎10'℞	Exact
--- □ ♀/♂	11-20-1999	05:46 am	Asc □ ♀/♂	Ar-Na	22°♊08'	22°♓08'	Exact
☉ - □ ♀/☊	11-28-1999	05:20 am	☉ □ ♀/☊	Ar-Na	27°♊55'	27°♓55'	Exact
♆ — ⚻ ☽	11-28-1999	12:59 pm	♆ ⚻ ☽	Tr-Na	02°♒10'	17°♊10'	Exact
♂ -- ⚻ ☽	11-28-1999	09:40 pm	♂ ⚻ ☽	Tr-Na	02°♒10'	17°♊10'	Exact
♅ — ☌ Mc	11-28-1999	10:51 pm	♅ ☌ Mc	Tr-Na	13°♒26'	13°♒26'	Exact
♄ -- ⚻ ☉/♆	11-30-1999	02:34 am	♄ ⚻ ☉/♆	Ar-Na	19°♐10'	04°♌10'	Exact
♂ -- □ ♄	12-03-1999	03:10 am	♂ □ ♄	Tr-Na	05°♒24'	05°♏24'℞	Exact
♂ -- □ Asc	12-07-1999	00:37 am	♂ □ Asc	Tr-Na	08°♒24'	08°♉24'	Exact
♂ -- □ ☿	12-08-1999	06:29 pm	♂ □ ☿	Tr-Na	09°♒45'	09°♉45'	Exact
♂ -- ⚻ ♃	12-10-1999	11:51 am	♂ ⚻ ♃	Tr-Na	11°♒05'	26°♊05'	Exact
♄ -- ∠ ♃	12-13-1999	10:08 am	♄ ∠ ♃	Tr-Na	11°♉05'℞	26°♊05'	Exact
♂ -- ☌ Mc	12-13-1999	01:00 pm	♂ ☌ Mc	Tr-Na	13°♒26'	13°♒26'	Exact
♂ -- □ ☉	12-14-1999	11:44 am	♂ □ ☉	Tr-Na	14°♒10'	14°♉10'	Exact
♅ — □ ☉	12-18-1999	03:29 pm	♅ □ ☉	Tr-Na	14°♒10'	14°♉10'	Exact
♃ -- SD	12-20-1999	09:42 am	♃ SD	Tr-Na	25°♈01'		
♂ -- ∠ ♂	12-24-1999	02:07 am	♂ ∠ ♂	Tr-Na	21°♒36'	06°♑36'	Exact
♂ -- ☍ ♇	12-25-1999	06:58 am	♂ ☍ ♇	Tr-Na	22°♒32'	22°♌32'	Exact
☊ — □ ♄	12-25-1999	10:30 am	☊ □ ♄	Tr-Na	05°♌24'℞	05°♏24'℞	Exact
♂ -- ∠ ☊	01-08-2000	00:06 am	♂ ∠ ☊	Tr-Na	03°♓10'	18°♑10'℞	Exact
♂ -- ⚻ ♅	01-09-2000	09:50 pm	♂ ⚻ ♅	Tr-Na	04°♓39'	19°♋39'	Exact
♄ -- SD	01-11-2000	11:19 pm	♄ SD	Tr-Na	10°♉17'		
♂ -- □ ♀	01-13-2000	07:35 pm	♂ □ ♀	Tr-Na	07°♓40'	07°♊40'	Exact
♂ -- ⚻ ♆	01-15-2000	05:49 pm	♂ ⚻ ♆	Tr-Na	09°♓10'	24°♎10'℞	Exact
☽ □ Asc	01-16-2000	01:15 am	☽ □ Asc	Pr-Na	08°♒24'	08°♉24'	Exact
♂ -- □ ☽	01-26-2000	02:18 am	♂ □ ☽	Tr-Na	17°♓10'	17°♊10'	Exact
♂ -- ⚻ ♄	01-30-2000	07:31 am	♂ ⚻ ♄	Tr-Na	20°♓24'	05°♏24'℞	Exact
♂ -- ∠ Asc	02-03-2000	05:11 am	♂ ∠ Asc	Tr-Na	23°♓24'	08°♉24'	Exact
♂ -- ∠ ☿	02-04-2000	11:16 pm	♂ ∠ ☿	Tr-Na	24°♓45'	09°♉45'	Exact
♂ -- □ ♃	02-06-2000	04:57 pm	♂ □ ♃	Tr-Na	26°♓05'	26°♊05'	Exact
♂ -- ∠ Mc	02-09-2000	06:52 pm	♂ ∠ Mc	Tr-Na	28°♓26'	13°♒26'	Exact
♄ -- ∠ ♃	02-10-2000	06:53 am	♄ ∠ ♃	Tr-Na	11°♉05'	26°♊05'	Exact
♂ -- ∠ ☉	02-10-2000	05:52 pm	♂ ∠ ☉	Tr-Na	29°♓10'	14°♉10'	Exact
♂ -- □ ♂	02-20-2000	12:29 pm	♂ □ ♂	Tr-Na	06°♈36'	06°♑36'	Exact
♂ -- ⚻ ♇	02-21-2000	06:01 pm	♂ ⚻ ♇	Tr-Na	07°♈32'	22°♌32'	Exact

"Corinne" Time Flow

Aspect	Date	Time	Event	Type	P1 Pos.	P2 Pos	E/X/L
☽ □ ☿	02-22-2000	07:12 am	☽ □ ☿	Pr-Na	09°♒45'	09°♉45'	Exact
☊ --- ∠ ☽	02-24-2000	05:47 pm	☊ ∠ ☽	Tr-Na	02°♌10'℞	17°♊10'	Exact
♃ -- ∠ ☽	02-27-2000	01:32 am	♃ ∠ ☽	Tr-Na	02°♉10'	17°♊10'	Exact
♆ ---- □ ♄	03-02-2000	00:45 am	♆ □ ♄	Tr-Na	05°♒24'	05°♏24'℞	Exact
♇ ---- ∠ ♀/♄	03-03-2000	12:00 pm	♇ ∠ ♀/♄	Ar-Na	06°♎32'	21°♌32'	Exact
☽ ⚼ ☉/☊	03-04-2000	06:30 am	☽ ⚼ ☉/☊	Ar-Na	01°♌10'	16°♓10'	Exact
♆ ---- □ ☿/♂	03-04-2000	10:55 pm	♆ □ ☿/♂	Ar-Na	08°♐11'	08°♓11'	Exact
♂ -- □ ☊	03-06-2000	09:25 pm	♂ □ ☊	Tr-Na	18°♈10'	18°♑10'℞	Exact
♂ -- □ ♅	03-08-2000	08:54 pm	♂ □ ♅	Tr-Na	19°♈39'	19°♋39'	Exact
♄ -- □ Mc	03-12-2000	06:52 am	♄ □ Mc	Tr-Na	13°♉26'	13°♒26'	Exact
♂ -- ∠ ♀	03-12-2000	10:29 pm	♂ ∠ ♀	Tr-Na	22°♈40'	07°♊40'	Exact
♃ -- ☍ ♄	03-14-2000	11:24 am	♃ ☍ ♄	Tr-Na	05°♉24'	05°♏24'℞	Exact
♂ -- ☍ ♆	03-14-2000	10:43 pm	♂ ☍ ♆	Tr-Na	24°♈10'	24°♎10'℞	Exact
♇ ---- SR	03-15-2000	02:15 am	♇ SR	Tr-Na	12°♐54'℞		
♄ -- ☌ ☉	03-19-2000	02:21 pm	♄ ☌ ☉	Tr-Na	14°♉10'	14°♉10'	Exact
♂ -- ☍ ☽/♆	03-24-2000	06:50 am	♂ ☍ ☽/♆	Ar-Na	20°♒40'	20°♌40'	Exact
♂ -- ∠ ☽	03-25-2000	07:03 pm	♂ ∠ ☽	Tr-Na	02°♉10'	17°♊10'	Exact
♇ ---- □ ♂	03-27-2000	04:27 am	♇ □ ♂	Ar-Na	06°♎36'	06°♑36'	Exact
♃ -- ☌ Asc	03-28-2000	08:21 am	♃ ☌ Asc	Tr-Na	08°♉24'	08°♉24'	Exact
--- □ ♃/Asc	03-28-2000	11:02 am	☊ □ ♃/Asc	Ar-Na	02°♓15'	02°♊15'	Exact
♂ -- ☍ ♄	03-30-2000	05:37 am	♂ ☍ ♄	Tr-Na	05°♉24'	05°♏24'℞	Exact
♃ -- ☌ ☿	04-03-2000	07:49 am	♃ ☌ ☿	Tr-Na	09°♉45'	09°♉45'	Exact
♂ -- ☌ Asc	04-03-2000	08:28 am	♂ ☌ Asc	Tr-Na	08°♉24'	08°♉24'	Exact
♂ -- ☌ ☿	04-05-2000	04:57 am	♂ ☌ ☿	Tr-Na	09°♉45'	09°♉45'	Exact
♂ -- ∠ ♃	04-07-2000	01:03 am	♂ ∠ ♃	Tr-Na	11°♉05'	26°♊05'	Exact
♃ -- ∠ ♃	04-09-2000	03:14 am	♃ ∠ ♃	Tr-Na	11°♉05'	26°♊05'	Exact
♂ -- □ Mc	04-10-2000	07:21 am	♂ □ Mc	Tr-Na	13°♉26'	13°♒26'	Exact
♂ -- ☌ ☉	04-11-2000	07:45 am	♂ ☌ ☉	Tr-Na	14°♉10'	14°♉10'	Exact
☽ ☌ ♆/Asc	04-17-2000	04:54 pm	☽ ☌ ♆/Asc	Ar-Na	01°♌17'	01°♌17'	Exact
♃ -- □ Mc	04-19-2000	05:43 am	♃ □ Mc	Tr-Na	13°♉26'	13°♒26'	Exact
♂ -- ⚼ ♂	04-21-2000	05:08 pm	♂ ⚼ ♂	Tr-Na	21°♉36'	06°♑36'	Exact
♃ -- ☌ ☉	04-22-2000	08:18 am	♃ ☌ ☉	Tr-Na	14°♉10'	14°♉10'	Exact
♂ -- □ ♇	04-23-2000	00:35 am	♂ □ ♇	Tr-Na	22°♉32'	22°♌32'	Exact
--- ∠ ☿/♄	05-06-2000	12:52 pm	Asc ∠ ☿/♄	Ar-Na	22°♊35'	07°♌35'	Exact
♆ ---- SR	05-08-2000	02:36 am	♆ SR	Tr-Na	06°♒34'℞		
♂ -- ⚼ ☊	05-08-2000	02:54 am	♂ ⚼ ☊	Tr-Na	03°♊10'	18°♑10'℞	Exact
♂ -- ∠ ♅	05-10-2000	05:41 am	♂ ∠ ♅	Tr-Na	04°♊39'	19°♋39'	Exact
♂ -- ☌ ♀	05-14-2000	02:09 pm	♂ ☌ ♀	Tr-Na	07°♊40'	07°♊40'	Exact
♂ -- ⚼ ♆	05-16-2000	05:48 pm	♂ ⚼ ♆	Tr-Na	09°♊10'	24°♎10'℞	Exact
♄ -- ⚼ ♂	05-19-2000	03:46 pm	♄ ⚼ ♂	Tr-Na	21°♉36'	06°♑36'	Exact
♃ -- ⚼ ♂	05-23-2000	04:22 pm	♃ ⚼ ♂	Tr-Na	21°♉36'	06°♑36'	Exact
♅ ---- SR	05-25-2000	00:01 am	♅ SR	Tr-Na	20°♒49'℞		
♄ -- □ ♇	05-26-2000	11:22 pm	♄ □ ♇	Tr-Na	22°♉32'	22°♌32'	Exact
♃ -- □ ♇	05-27-2000	03:45 pm	♃ □ ♇	Tr-Na	22°♉32'	22°♌32'	Exact
♂ -- ☌ ☽	05-28-2000	08:42 am	♂ ☌ ☽	Tr-Na	17°♊10'	17°♊10'	Exact
♀ - ∠ ♅/♆	05-28-2000	10:53 pm	♀ ∠ ♅/♆	Ar-Na	21°♋54'	06°♍54'	Exact
♂ -- ⚼ ♄	06-02-2000	02:53 am	♂ ⚼ ♄	Tr-Na	20°♊24'	05°♏24'℞	Exact
☽ ☌ Mc	06-03-2000	01:07 am	☽ ☌ Mc	Pr-Na	13°♒26'	13°♒26'	Exact
♂ -- ∠ Asc	06-06-2000	12:47 pm	♂ ∠ Asc	Tr-Na	23°♊24'	08°♉24'	Exact
♂ -- ∠ ☿	06-08-2000	12:27 pm	♂ ∠ ☿	Tr-Na	24°♊45'	09°♉45'	Exact
♅ ---- ∠ ♅/☊	06-09-2000	03:40 am	♅ ∠ ♅/☊	Ar-Na	03°♍55'	18°♎55'	Exact
♂ -- ☌ ♃	06-10-2000	11:42 am	♂ ☌ ♃	Tr-Na	26°♊05'	26°♊05'	Exact
☉ - ⚼ Mc	06-11-2000	01:03 pm	☉ ⚼ Mc	Ar-Na	28°♊26'	13°♒26'	Exact
♂ -- ⚼ Mc	06-13-2000	11:36 pm	♂ ⚼ Mc	Tr-Na	28°♊26'	13°♒26'	Exact
♂ -- ∠ ☉	06-15-2000	01:44 am	♂ ∠ ☉	Tr-Na	29°♊10'	14°♉10'	Exact
☽ □ ☉	06-23-2000	04:50 am	☽ □ ☉	Pr-Na	14°♒10'	14°♉10'	Exact
♂ -- ☍ ♂	06-26-2000	04:33 am	♂ ☍ ♂	Tr-Na	06°♋36'	06°♑36'	Exact
♂ -- ∠ ♇	06-27-2000	02:10 pm	♂ ∠ ♇	Tr-Na	07°♋32'	22°♌32'	Exact
☿ - ∠ ☿/Asc	07-04-2000	10:44 am	☿ ∠ ☿/Asc	Ar-Na	24°♊05'	09°♉05'	Exact
♂ -- ☍ ☊	07-13-2000	04:44 pm	♂ ☍ ☊	Tr-Na	18°♋10'	18°♑10'℞	Exact
♂ -- ☌ ♅	07-15-2000	10:49 pm	♂ ☌ ♅	Tr-Na	19°♋39'	19°♋39'	Exact
♃ -- ⚼ ☊	07-16-2000	00:27 am	♃ ⚼ ☊	Tr-Na	03°♊10'	18°♑10'℞	Exact
♆ ---- □ ♄	07-19-2000	07:35 am	♆ □ ♄	Tr-Na	05°♒24'℞	05°♏24'℞	Exact

diruption, change of tactic

♂ ♃☌☉

SP☽☌MC

"Corinne" Time Flow (Cont'd)

Aspect	Date	Time	Event	Type	P1 Pos.	P2 Pos	E/X/L
♂ -- ∠ ♀	07-20-2000	01:56 pm	♂ ∠ ♀	Tr-Na	22°♋40'	07°♊40'	Exact
♂ -- □ ♆	07-22-2000	08:49 pm	♂ □ ♆	Tr-Na	24°♋10'	24°♎10'℞	Exact
♃ -- ∠ ♅	07-24-2000	02:50 am	♃ ∠ ♅	Tr-Na	04°♊39'	19°♋39'	Exact
☊ --- □ ♆	07-24-2000	05:15 pm	☊ □ ♆	Tr-Na	24°♋10'℞	24°♎10'℞	Exact
☽ □ ♅/Mc	07-24-2000	07:47 pm	☽ □ ♅/Mc	Ar-Na	01°♌32'	01°♉32'	Exact
♂ -- ∠ ☽	08-04-2000	04:28 am	♂ ∠ ☽	Tr-Na	02°♌10'	17°♊10'	Exact
♂ -- □ ♄	08-09-2000	05:12 am	♂ □ ♄	Tr-Na	05°♌24'	05°♏24'℞	Exact
♃ -- ☌ ♀	08-12-2000	06:33 am	♃ ☌ ♀	Tr-Na	07°♊40'	07°♊40'	Exact
♂ -- □ Asc	08-13-2000	09:03 pm	♂ □ Asc	Tr-Na	08°♌24'	08°♉24'	Exact
♂ -- □ ☿	08-15-2000	11:20 pm	♂ □ ☿	Tr-Na	09°♌45'	09°♉45'	Exact
♂ -- ∠ ♃	08-18-2000	01:08 am	♂ ∠ ♃	Tr-Na	11°♌05'	26°♊05'	Exact
♇ ---- SD	08-20-2000	12:06 pm	♇ SD	Tr-Na	10°♐09'		
♂ -- ☍ Mc	08-21-2000	05:26 pm	♂ ☍ Mc	Tr-Na	13°♌26'	13°♒26'	Exact
☊ --- ∠ ♀	08-21-2000	09:10 pm	☊ ∠ ♀	Tr-Na	22°♋40'℞	07°♊40'	Exact
♂ -- □ ☉	08-22-2000	08:56 pm	♂ □ ☉	Tr-Na	14°♌10'	14°♉10'	Exact
♃ -- ⚼ ♆	08-24-2000	06:04 am	♃ ⚼ ♆	Tr-Na	09°♊10'	24°♎10'℞	Exact
♂ -- ⚼ ♂	09-03-2000	12:56 pm	♂ ⚼ ♂	Tr-Na	21°♌36'	06°♑36'	Exact
--- ☌ ♀/☊	09-03-2000	01:07 pm	Mc ☌ ♀/☊	Ar-Na	27°♓55'	27°♓55'	Exact
♂ -- ☌ ♇	09-05-2000	00:09 am	♂ ☌ ♇	Tr-Na	22°♌32'	22°♌32'	Exact
☉ - ☌ ♀/♅	09-05-2000	10:30 pm	☉ ☌ ♀/♅	Ar-Na	28°♊40'	28°♊40'	Exact
♄ -- SR	09-12-2000	05:52 am	♄ SR	Tr-Na	00°♊59'℞		
♂ -- ⚼ ☊	09-21-2000	07:59 pm	♂ ⚼ ☊	Tr-Na	03°♍10'	18°♑10'℞	Exact
♂ -- ∠ ♅	09-24-2000	04:18 am	♂ ∠ ♅	Tr-Na	04°♍39'	19°♋39'	Exact
♂ -- □ ♀	09-28-2000	11:55 pm	♂ □ ♀	Tr-Na	07°♍40'	07°♊40'	Exact
♃ -- SR	09-29-2000	07:46 am	♃ SR	Tr-Na	11°♊14'℞		
♂ -- ∠ ♆	10-01-2000	08:58 am	♂ ∠ ♆	Tr-Na	09°♍10'	24°♎10'℞	Exact
♇ ---- ☍ ♃/☊	10-13-2000	05:32 am	♇ ☍ ♃/☊	Ar-Na	07°♎07'	07°♈07'	Exact
♂ -- □ ☽	10-14-2000	04:00 am	♂ □ ☽	Tr-Na	17°♍10'	17°♊10'	Exact
♆ ---- SD	10-15-2000	04:49 am	♆ SD	Tr-Na	03°♒47'		
☊ --- ☌ ♅	10-18-2000	01:02 am	☊ ☌ ♅	Tr-Na	19°♋39'℞	19°♋39'	Exact
♂ -- ∠ ♄	10-19-2000	09:11 am	♂ ∠ ♄	Tr-Na	20°♍24'	05°♏24'℞	Exact
♂ -- ⚼ Asc	10-24-2000	05:02 am	♂ ⚼ Asc	Tr-Na	23°♍24'	08°♉24'	Exact
♅ ---- SD	10-26-2000	06:54 am	♅ SD	Tr-Na	16°♒54'		
♂ -- ⚼ ☿	10-26-2000	09:06 am	♂ ⚼ ☿	Tr-Na	24°♍45'	09°♉45'	Exact
♂ -- □ ♃	10-28-2000	12:40 pm	♂ □ ♃	Tr-Na	26°♍05'	26°♊05'	Exact
☉ - □ ☉/Mc	10-29-2000	05:02 pm	☉ □ ☉/Mc	Ar-Na	28°♊48'	28°♓48'	Exact
♂ -- ⚼ Mc	11-01-2000	08:07 am	♂ ⚼ Mc	Tr-Na	28°♍26'	13°♒26'	Exact
♂ -- ⚼ ☉	11-02-2000	12:35 pm	♂ ⚼ ☉	Tr-Na	29°♍10'	14°♉10'	Exact
♃ -- ⚼ ♆	11-04-2000	04:22 am	♃ ⚼ ♆	Tr-Na	09°♊10'℞	24°♎10'℞	Exact
☿ - ☍ ♄/Mc	11-13-2000	05:00 am	☿ ☍ ♄/Mc	Ar-Na	24°♊25'	24°♐25'	Exact
♂ -- □ ♂	11-14-2000	02:50 pm	♂ □ ♂	Tr-Na	06°♎36'	06°♑36'	Exact
☊ --- ☍ ☊	11-14-2000	10:28 pm	☊ ☍ ☊	Tr-Na	18°♋10'℞	18°♑10'	Exact
♂ -- ∠ ♇	11-16-2000	03:21 am	♂ ∠ ♇	Tr-Na	07°♎32'	22°♌32'	Exact
♃ -- ☌ ♀	11-16-2000	01:16 pm	♃ ☌ ♀	Tr-Na	07°♊40'℞	07°♊40'	Exact
☽ ∠ ♀/♃	11-30-2000	07:31 am	☽ ∠ ♀/♃	Ar-Na	01°♌53'	16°♊53'	Exact
♂ -- □ ☊	12-03-2000	03:00 pm	♂ □ ☊	Tr-Na	18°♎10'	18°♑10'℞	Exact
♂ -- □ ♅	12-06-2000	01:46 am	♂ □ ♅	Tr-Na	19°♎39'	19°♋39'	Exact
♃ -- ∠ ♅	12-09-2000	02:22 am	♃ ∠ ♅	Tr-Na	04°♊39'℞	19°♋39'	Exact
--- □ ☿/♃	12-10-2000	09:17 pm	☊ □ ☿/♃	Ar-Na	02°♓55'	02°♊55'	Exact
♂ -- ⚼ ♀	12-11-2000	02:37 am	♂ ⚼ ♀	Tr-Na	22°♎40'	07°♊40'	Exact
☽ ∠ ☉/♅	12-11-2000	11:48 pm	☽ ∠ ☉/♅	Ar-Na	01°♌54'	16°♊54'	Exact
♂ -- ☌ ♆	12-13-2000	02:22 pm	♂ ☌ ♆	Tr-Na	24°♎10'	24°♎10'℞	Exact
♃ -- ⚼ ☊	12-21-2000	10:30 am	♃ ⚼ ☊	Tr-Na	03°♊10'℞	18°♑10'℞	Exact
♂ -- ⚼ ☽	12-27-2000	01:26 am	♂ ⚼ ☽	Tr-Na	02°♏10'	17°♊10'	Exact
☽ ☌ ☿/♆	12-31-2000	03:11 am	☽ ☌ ☿/♆	Ar-Na	01°♌57'	01°♌57'	Exact
♂ -- ☌ ♄	01-01-2001	02:14 pm	♂ ☌ ♄	Tr-Na	05°♏24'	05°♏24'℞	Exact
☉ - □ ♄/♇	01-02-2001	10:58 am	☉ □ ♄/♇	Ar-Na	28°♊58'	28°♍58'	Exact
♆ ---- □ ♄	01-03-2001	00:36 am	♆ □ ♄	Tr-Na	05°♒24'	05°♏24'℞	Exact
♂ -- ☍ Asc	01-06-2001	05:53 pm	♂ ☍ Asc	Tr-Na	08°♏24'	08°♉24'	Exact
♂ -- ☍ ☿	01-09-2001	01:41 am	♂ ☍ ☿	Tr-Na	09°♏45'	09°♉45'	Exact
♂ -- ⚼ ♃	01-11-2001	09:06 am	♂ ⚼ ♃	Tr-Na	11°♏05'	26°♊05'	Exact
♀ - ⚼ ♂/Asc	01-12-2001	10:32 am	♀ ⚼ ♂/Asc	Ar-Na	22°♋30'	07°♓30'	Exact

"Corinne" Time Flow (Cont'd)

Aspect	Date	Time	Event	Type	P1 Pos.	P2 Pos	E/X/L
♂ -- □ Mc	01-15-2001	11:47 am	♂ □ Mc	Tr-Na	13°♏26'	13°♒26'	Exact
♂ -- ☍ ☉	01-16-2001	06:37 pm	♂ ☍ ☉	Tr-Na	14°♏10'	14°♉10'	Exact
♄ -- SD	01-24-2001	06:18 pm	♄ SD	Tr-Na	24°♉04'		
♃ -- SD	01-25-2001	03:04 am	♃ SD	Tr-Na	01°♊11'		
♂ -- ∠ ♂	01-30-2001	00:49 am	♂ ∠ ♂	Tr-Na	21°♏36'	06°♑36'	Exact
♂ -- □ ♇	01-31-2001	05:28 pm	♂ □ ♇	Tr-Na	22°♏32'	22°♌32'	Exact
☽ ☍ ♇	02-07-2001	02:31 am	☽ ☍ ♇	Pr-Na	22°♒32'	22°♌32'	Exact
♂ -- ∠ ☊	02-20-2001	06:02 pm	♂ ∠ ☊	Tr-Na	03°♐10'	18°♑10'℞	Exact
♅ ---- ∠ ♂	02-22-2001	09:58 pm	♅ ∠ ♂	Tr-Na	21°♒36'	06°♑36'	Exact
♂ -- ☍ ♀/♄	02-23-2001	04:37 am	♂ ☍ ♀/♄	Ar-Na	21°♒32'	21°♌32'	Exact
♂ -- ⚻ ♅	02-23-2001	03:56 pm	♂ ⚻ ♅	Tr-Na	04°♐39'	19°♋39'	Exact
♄ -- ∠ ♇/☊	02-26-2001	00:23 am	♄ ∠ ♇/☊	Ar-Na	20°♐21'	05°♏21'	Exact
--- □ ♆/♇	02-26-2001	00:54 am	Asc □ ♆/♇	Ar-Na	23°♊21'	23°♍21'	Exact
♃ -- ⚻ ☊	03-01-2001	00:42 am	♃ ⚻ ☊	Tr-Na	03°♊10'	18°♑10'℞	Exact
♂ -- ☍ ♀	03-01-2001	06:34 pm	♂ ☍ ♀	Tr-Na	07°♐40'	07°♊40'	Exact
♂ -- ∠ ♆	03-04-2001	08:44 pm	♂ ∠ ♆	Tr-Na	09°♐10'	24°♎10'℞	Exact
♅ ---- ☍ ♇	03-11-2001	09:05 pm	♅ ☍ ♇	Tr-Na	22°♒32'	22°♌32'	Exact
♃ -- ∠ ♅	03-12-2001	10:48 pm	♃ ∠ ♅	Tr-Na	04°♊39'	19°♋39'	Exact
♇ ---- SR	03-17-2001	04:49 pm	♇ SR	Tr-Na	15°♐17'℞		
♇ ---- ∠ ♇	03-18-2001	09:07 pm	♇ ∠ ♇	Ar-Na	07°♎32'	22°♌32'	Exact
☽ ∠ ☽	03-18-2001	09:07 pm	☽ ∠ ☽	Ar-Na	02°♌10'	17°♊10'	Exact
♀ - ∠ ♀	03-18-2001	09:07 pm	♀ ∠ ♀	Ar-Na	22°♋40'	07°♊40'	Exact
☉ - ∠ ☉	03-18-2001	09:07 pm	☉ ∠ ☉	Ar-Na	29°♊10'	14°♉10'	Exact
☿ - ∠ ☿	03-18-2001	09:07 pm	☿ ∠ ☿	Ar-Na	24°♊45'	09°♉45'	Exact
♂ -- ∠ ♂	03-18-2001	09:07 pm	♂ ∠ ♂	Ar-Na	21°♒36'	06°♑36'	Exact
Asc ---- ∠ Asc	03-18-2001	09:07 pm	Asc ∠ Asc	Ar-Na	23°♊24'	08°♉24'	Exact
♃ -- ∠ ♃	03-18-2001	09:07 pm	♃ ∠ ♃	Ar-Na	11°♌05'	26°♊05'	Exact
♄ -- ∠ ♄	03-18-2001	09:07 pm	♄ ∠ ♄	Ar-Na	20°♐24'	05°♏24'℞	Exact
♅ ---- ∠ ♅	03-18-2001	09:07 pm	♅ ∠ ♅	Ar-Na	04°♍39'	19°♋39'	Exact
♆ ---- ∠ ♆	03-18-2001	09:07 pm	♆ ∠ ♆	Ar-Na	09°♐10'	24°♎10'℞	Exact
☊ ---- ∠ ☊	03-18-2001	09:07 pm	☊ ∠ ☊	Ar-Na	03°♓10'	18°♑10'℞	Exact
Mc ---- ∠ Mc	03-18-2001	09:07 pm	Mc ∠ Mc	Ar-Na	28°♓26'	13°♒26'	Exact
♂ -- ☍ ☽	03-22-2001	06:01 pm	♂ ☍ ☽	Tr-Na	17°♐10'	17°♊10'	Exact
♂ -- ∠ ♄	03-31-2001	01:38 am	♂ ∠ ♄	Tr-Na	20°♐24'	05°♏24'℞	Exact

"Corinne" Time Flow (Cont'd)

a wistful hope for intimacy leading to love, and perhaps some other dimension of compulsion.

As soon as the trip was underway, there were tensions. Negative animus and anima manifestations abounded. The scapegoat "reason" provided by Corrine was Ian's *snoring!* This was certainly a displacement of the real problems she had being with Ian. She criticized him terribly, daily, and added other "whammies" to the package as well.

Ian tried so hard to make things work and actually had an operation to correct the snoring condition, but the operation was not successful. In the end, Ian simply said, "I can't take any more criticism." Of course, the criticism led to rejection, and finally to abandonment.

Aspect	Date	Time	Event	Type	P1 Pos.	P2 Pos	E/X/L
♂ -- ☍ ☉	03-07-2000	11:07 am	♂ ☍ ☉	Tr-Na	18°♈36'	18°♎36'	Exact
♂ -- □ ♃	03-13-2000	04:09 pm	♂ □ ♃	Tr-Na	23°♈13'	23°♑13'	Exact
♇ ---- SR	03-15-2000	02:15 am	♇ SR	Tr-Na	12°♐54'℞		
♅ ---- ⚼ ☿	03-16-2000	01:05 pm	♅ ⚼ ☿	Tr-Na	18°♒58'	03°♎58'℞	Exact
♂ -- ⚼ Asc	03-21-2000	02:15 pm	♂ ⚼ Asc	Tr-Na	29°♈05'	14°♐05'	Exact
♂ -- ⚼ ♄	03-22-2000	01:13 am	♂ ⚼ ♄	Tr-Na	29°♈25'	14°♍25'	Exact
♂ -- ∠ ☽	03-22-2000	04:07 pm	♂ ∠ ☽	Tr-Na	29°♈52'	14°♊52'	Exact
♄ -- ∠ ☉/♂	03-25-2000	11:59 pm	♄ ∠ ☉/♂	Ar-Na	05°♏01'	20°♍01'	Exact
☊ --- ∠ ☽	04-08-2000	00:20 am	☊ ∠ ☽	Tr-Na	29°♋52'℞	14°♊52'	Exact
♅ ---- ⚼ ♅	04-10-2000	06:22 am	♅ ⚼ ♅	Tr-Na	20°♒01'	05°♋01'℞	Exact
♂ -- □ ♇	04-16-2000	11:06 am	♂ □ ♇	Tr-Na	17°♉51'	17°♌51'	Exact
☊ --- ∠ ♄	04-16-2000	03:24 pm	☊ ∠ ♄	Tr-Na	29°♋25'℞	14°♍25'	Exact
♂ -- ⚼ ☿	04-18-2000	00:33 am	♂ ⚼ ☿	Tr-Na	18°♉58'	03°♎58'℞	Exact
☽ □ ♃/♇	04-18-2000	01:08 am	☽ □ ♃/♇	Ar-Na	05°♌32'	05°♏32'	Exact
♂ -- ∠ ♅	04-19-2000	11:45 am	♂ ∠ ♅	Tr-Na	20°♉01'	05°♋01'℞	Exact
♄ -- □ ♇	04-20-2000	08:43 am	♄ □ ♇	Tr-Na	17°♉51'	17°♌51'	Exact
♂ -- □ ♂	04-21-2000	11:36 am	♂ □ ♂	Tr-Na	21°♉26'	21°♌26'	Exact
☊ --- ⚼ Asc	04-22-2000	11:41 pm	☊ ⚼ Asc	Tr-Na	29°♋05'℞	14°♐05'	Exact
♅ ---- □ ♅/☊	04-23-2000	02:12 pm	♅ □ ♅/☊	Ar-Na	25°♌42'	25°♉42'	Exact
♂ -- □ Mc	04-28-2000	10:13 pm	♂ □ Mc	Tr-Na	26°♉43'	26°♌43'	Exact
♄ -- ⚼ ☿	04-29-2000	04:22 am	♄ ⚼ ☿	Tr-Na	18°♉58'	03°♎58'℞	Exact
♂ -- ⚼ ♆	05-03-2000	04:06 pm	♂ ⚼ ♆	Tr-Na	00°♊03'	15°♎03'	Exact
♂ -- ∠ ☊	05-05-2000	01:46 pm	♂ ∠ ☊	Tr-Na	01°♊23'	16°♈23'℞	Exact
♂ -- ☍ ♀	05-06-2000	02:38 pm	♂ ☍ ♀	Tr-Na	02°♊07'	02°♐07'	Exact
♄ -- ∠ ♅	05-07-2000	08:13 am	♄ ∠ ♅	Tr-Na	20°♉01'	05°♋01'℞	Exact
♃ -- □ ♇	05-07-2000	08:59 pm	♃ □ ♇	Tr-Na	17°♉51'	17°♌51'	Exact
♆ ---- SR	05-08-2000	02:36 am	♆ SR	Tr-Na	06°♒34'℞		
♂ -- ⚼ ☉	05-08-2000	05:33 pm	♂ ⚼ ☉	Tr-Na	03°♊36'	18°♎36'	Exact
♆ ---- ⚼ ☽/Mc	05-12-2000	01:10 pm	♆ ⚼ ☽/Mc	Ar-Na	05°♐47'	20°♋47'	Exact
♃ -- ⚼ ☿	05-12-2000	01:29 pm	♃ ⚼ ☿	Tr-Na	18°♉58'	03°♎58'℞	Exact
♂ -- ⚼ ♃	05-15-2000	09:04 am	♂ ⚼ ♃	Tr-Na	08°♊13'	23°♑13'	Exact
♃ -- ∠ ♅	05-16-2000	11:21 pm	♃ ∠ ♅	Tr-Na	20°♉01'	05°♋01'℞	Exact
♄ -- □ ♂	05-18-2000	09:06 am	♄ □ ♂	Tr-Na	21°♉26'	21°♌26'	Exact
♃ -- □ ♂	05-22-2000	11:40 pm	♃ □ ♂	Tr-Na	21°♉26'	21°♌26'	Exact
♂ -- ☍ Asc	05-23-2000	08:43 pm	♂ ☍ Asc	Tr-Na	14°♊05'	14°♐05'	Exact
♂ -- □ ♄	05-24-2000	08:27 am	♂ □ ♄	Tr-Na	14°♊25'	14°♍25'	Exact
♅ ---- SR	05-25-2000	00:01 am	♅ SR	Tr-Na	20°♒49'℞		
♂ -- ☌ ☽	05-25-2000	00:26 am	♂ ☌ ☽	Tr-Na	14°♊52'	14°♊52'	Exact
--- □ ☉/☊	05-27-2000	09:44 pm	Mc □ ☉/☊	Ar-Na	17°♎30'	17°♑30'	Exact
♃ -- □ Mc	06-14-2000	09:50 pm	♃ □ Mc	Tr-Na	26°♉43'	26°♌43'	Exact
♂ -- ∠ ♇	06-20-2000	01:47 pm	♂ ∠ ♇	Tr-Na	02°♋51'	17°♌51'	Exact
♂ -- □ ☿	06-22-2000	05:50 am	♂ □ ☿	Tr-Na	03°♋58'	03°♎58'℞	Exact
♂ -- ☌ ♅	06-23-2000	07:29 pm	♂ ☌ ♅	Tr-Na	05°♋01'	05°♋01'℞	Exact
♃ -- □ Asc	06-23-2000	08:16 pm	♃ □ Asc	Ar-Na	14°♓05'	14°♐05'	Exact
♆ ---- ☌ ☉/♃	06-24-2000	04:20 am	♆ ☌ ☉/♃	Ar-Na	05°♐55'	05°♐55'	Exact
♂ -- ∠ ♂	06-25-2000	10:39 pm	♂ ∠ ♂	Tr-Na	06°♋26'	21°♌26'	Exact
♃ -- ⚼ ♆	06-30-2000	08:37 am	♃ ⚼ ♆	Tr-Na	00°♊03'	15°♎03'	Exact
♄ -- □ Mc	07-01-2000	10:46 am	♄ □ Mc	Tr-Na	26°♉43'	26°♌43'	Exact
♂ -- ∠ Mc	07-03-2000	09:24 pm	♂ ∠ Mc	Tr-Na	11°♋43'	26°♌43'	Exact
♃ -- ∠ ☊	07-06-2000	09:01 pm	♃ ∠ ☊	Tr-Na	01°♊23'	16°♈23'℞	Exact
♂ -- □ ♆	07-08-2000	10:54 pm	♂ □ ♆	Tr-Na	15°♋03'	15°♎03'	Exact
♃ -- ☍ ♀	07-10-2000	12:42 pm	♃ ☍ ♀	Tr-Na	02°♊07'	02°♐07'	Exact
♅ ---- ⚼ ♅	07-10-2000	01:33 pm	♅ ⚼ ♅	Tr-Na	20°♒01'℞	05°♋01'℞	Exact
♂ -- □ ☊	07-10-2000	11:36 pm	♂ □ ☊	Tr-Na	16°♋23'	16°♈23'℞	Exact
♂ -- ⚼ ♀	07-12-2000	02:06 am	♂ ⚼ ♀	Tr-Na	17°♋07'	02°♐07'	Exact
♂ -- □ ☉	07-14-2000	08:20 am	♂ □ ☉	Tr-Na	18°♋36'	18°♎36'	Exact
♃ -- ⚼ ☉	07-18-2000	07:13 am	♃ ⚼ ☉	Tr-Na	03°♊36'	18°♎36'	Exact
♂ -- ☍ ♃	07-21-2000	10:03 am	♂ ☍ ♃	Tr-Na	23°♋13'	23°♑13'	Exact
--- ⚼ ☉/♂	07-25-2000	01:23 am	Asc ⚼ ☉/♂	Ar-Na	05°♒01'	20°♍01'	Exact
♂ -- ⚼ Asc	07-30-2000	10:07 am	♂ ⚼ Asc	Tr-Na	29°♋05'	14°♐05'	Exact
♂ -- ∠ ♄	07-30-2000	10:34 pm	♂ ∠ ♄	Tr-Na	29°♋25'	14°♍25'	Exact
♂ -- ∠ ☽	07-31-2000	03:29 pm	♂ ∠ ☽	Tr-Na	29°♋52'	14°♊52'	Exact
♅ ---- ⚼ ☿	08-07-2000	09:22 pm	♅ ⚼ ☿	Tr-Na	18°♒58'℞	03°♎58'℞	Exact
♀ - ∠ ♀/Asc	08-08-2000	07:44 am	♀ ∠ ♀/Asc	Ar-Na	23°♑06'	08°♐06'	Exact
♄ -- ⚼ ♆	08-10-2000	07:48 pm	♄ ⚼ ♆	Tr-Na	00°♊03'	15°♎03'	Exact

♃= Asc ★

"Ian" Time Flow

Aspect	Date	Time	Event	Type	P1 Pos.	P2 Pos	E/X/L
☊ --- ☍ ♃	08-11-2000	01:17 pm	☊ ☍ ♃	Tr-Na	23°♋13'℞	23°♑13'	Exact
♃ -- Qd ♃	08-16-2000	08:38 am	♃ Qd ♃	Tr-Na	08°♊13'	23°♑13'	Exact
☿ - ∠ ♀/♇	08-19-2000	11:32 pm	☿ ∠ ♀/♇	Ar-Na	24°♏59'	09°♎59'	Exact
☽ ∠ ♆/Mc	08-20-2000	00:51 am	☽ ∠ ♆/Mc	Ar-Na	05°♌53'	20°♍53'	Exact
♇ ---- SD	08-20-2000	12:06 pm	♇ SD	Tr-Na	10°♐09'		
♃ -- Qd ♄/Asc	08-23-2000	08:54 am	♃ Qd ♄/Asc	Ar-Na	14°♓15'	29°♎15'	Exact
♂ -- ☌ ♇	08-28-2000	03:38 pm	♂ ☌ ♇	Tr-Na	17°♌51'	17°♌51'	Exact
♂ -- ∠ ☿	08-30-2000	09:39 am	♂ ∠ ☿	Tr-Na	18°♌58'	03°♎58'℞	Exact
--- ☌ ♂/Asc	08-31-2000	08:19 am	Mc ☌ ♂/Asc	Ar-Na	17°♎45'	17°♎45'	Exact
♂ -- ∠ ♅	09-01-2000	01:08 am	♂ ∠ ♅	Tr-Na	20°♌01'	05°♋01'℞	Exact
♂ -- ☌ ♂	09-03-2000	06:45 am	♂ ☌ ♂	Tr-Na	21°♌26'	21°♌26'	Exact
♅ ---- ☍ ♇	09-06-2000	00:47 am	♅ ☍ ♇	Tr-Na	17°♒51'℞	17°♌51'	Exact
☿ - □ ♅/♆	09-07-2000	07:09 am	☿ □ ♅/♆	Ar-Na	25°♏02'	25°♌02'	Exact
♂ -- ☌ Mc	09-11-2000	02:25 pm	♂ ☌ Mc	Tr-Na	26°♌43'	26°♌43'	Exact
♄ -- SR	09-12-2000	05:52 am	♄ SR	Tr-Na	00°♊59'℞		
♂ -- ∠ ♆	09-16-2000	09:19 pm	♂ ∠ ♆	Tr-Na	00°♍03'	15°♎03'	Exact
♂ -- Qd ☊	09-19-2000	00:06 am	♂ Qd ☊	Tr-Na	01°♍23'	16°♈23'℞	Exact
♂ -- □ ♀	09-20-2000	03:44 am	♂ □ ♀	Tr-Na	02°♍07'	02°♐07'	Exact
♂ -- ∠ ☉	09-22-2000	12:14 pm	♂ ∠ ☉	Tr-Na	03°♍36'	18°♎36'	Exact
♀ - ☌ ♃	09-22-2000	07:09 pm	♀ ☌ ♃	Ar-Na	23°♑13'	23°♑13'	Exact
♃ -- SR	09-29-2000	07:46 am	♃ SR	Tr-Na	11°♊14'℞		
♄ -- ☌ ♃/♇	09-29-2000	03:33 pm	♄ ☌ ♃/♇	Ar-Na	05°♏32'	05°♏32'	Exact
♂ -- Qd ♃	09-29-2000	08:50 pm	♂ Qd ♃	Tr-Na	08°♍13'	23°♑13'	Exact
♀ - □ ♀/♄	10-07-2000	08:19 pm	♀ □ ♀/♄	Ar-Na	23°♑16'	23°♎16'	Exact
♂ -- □ Asc	10-09-2000	05:20 am	♂ □ Asc	Tr-Na	14°♍05'	14°♐05'	Exact
♂ -- ☌ ♄	10-09-2000	06:15 pm	♂ ☌ ♄	Tr-Na	14°♍25'	14°♍25'	Exact
♂ -- □ ☽	10-10-2000	11:49 am	♂ □ ☽	Tr-Na	14°♍52'	14°♊52'	Exact
♄ -- Qd ♆	10-14-2000	08:59 pm	♄ Qd ♆	Tr-Na	00°♊03'℞	15°♎03'	Exact
♆ ---- SD	10-15-2000	04:49 am	♆ SD	Tr-Na	03°♒47'		
♃ -- ☍ ♄	10-22-2000	09:28 pm	♃ ☍ ♄	Ar-Na	14°♓25'	14°♍25'	Exact
♅ ---- SD	10-26-2000	06:54 am	♅ SD	Tr-Na	16°♒54'		
☿ - Qd ☿/☊	10-29-2000	04:29 am	☿ Qd ☿/☊	Ar-Na	25°♏11'	10°♋11'	Exact
--- ∠ ♂/♄	10-30-2000	08:53 pm	Mc ∠ ♂/♄	Ar-Na	17°♎56'	02°♍56'	Exact
♇ ---- ∠ ♂/Mc	11-02-2000	04:37 am	♇ ∠ ♂/Mc	Ar-Na	09°♎05'	24°♌05'	Exact
☊ --- □ ☉	11-06-2000	09:11 pm	☊ □ ☉	Tr-Na	18°♋36'℞	18°♎36'	Exact
♂ -- ∠ ♇	11-08-2000	12:19 pm	♂ ∠ ♇	Tr-Na	02°♎51'	17°♌51'	Exact
♂ -- ☌ ☿	11-10-2000	07:53 am	♂ ☌ ☿	Tr-Na	03°♎58'	03°♎58'℞	Exact
♂ -- □ ♅	11-12-2000	00:49 am	♂ □ ♅	Tr-Na	05°♎01'	05°♋01'℞	Exact
♃ -- Qd ♃	11-12-2000	06:06 am	♃ Qd ♃	Tr-Na	08°♊13'℞	23°♑13'	Exact
♃ -- ☍ ☽/Asc	11-13-2000	03:59 pm	♃ ☍ ☽/Asc	Ar-Na	14°♓28'	14°♍28'	Exact
♂ -- ∠ ♂	11-14-2000	08:25 am	♂ ∠ ♂	Tr-Na	06°♎26'	21°♌26'	Exact
♅ ---- ∠ ☉/☿	11-18-2000	08:15 pm	♅ ∠ ☉/☿	Ar-Na	26°♌17'	11°♎17'	Exact
♂ -- ∠ Mc	11-22-2000	11:32 pm	♂ ∠ Mc	Tr-Na	11°♎43'	26°♌43'	Exact
♂ -- ☌ ♆	11-28-2000	11:24 am	♂ ☌ ♆	Tr-Na	15°♎03'	15°♎03'	Exact
♄ -- □ Mc	11-28-2000	10:46 pm	♄ □ Mc	Tr-Na	26°♉43'℞	26°♌43'	Exact
♂ -- ☍ ☊	11-30-2000	04:16 pm	♂ ☍ ☊	Tr-Na	16°♎23'	16°♈23'℞	Exact
♂ -- ∠ ♀	12-01-2000	09:03 pm	♂ ∠ ♀	Tr-Na	17°♎07'	02°♐07'	Exact
♂ -- ☌ ☉	12-04-2000	07:57 am	♂ ☌ ☉	Tr-Na	18°♎36'	18°♎36'	Exact
☊ --- Qd ♀	12-04-2000	09:19 pm	☊ Qd ♀	Tr-Na	17°♋07'℞	02°♐07'	Exact
♂ -- □ ♃	12-12-2000	00:31 am	♂ □ ♃	Tr-Na	23°♎13'	23°♑13'	Exact
♅ ---- ☍ ♇	12-13-2000	02:25 pm	♅ ☍ ♇	Tr-Na	17°♒51'	17°♌51'	Exact
♃ -- Qd ☉	12-17-2000	03:01 pm	♃ Qd ☉	Tr-Na	03°♊36'℞	18°♎36'	Exact
☊ --- □ ☊	12-18-2000	02:12 pm	☊ □ ☊	Tr-Na	16°♋23'℞	16°♈23'℞	Exact
♂ -- ∠ Asc	12-21-2000	08:10 pm	♂ ∠ Asc	Tr-Na	29°♎05'	14°♐05'	Exact
♂ -- ∠ ♄	12-22-2000	09:47 am	♂ ∠ ♄	Tr-Na	29°♎25'	14°♍25'	Exact
♂ -- Qd ☽	12-23-2000	04:17 am	♂ Qd ☽	Tr-Na	29°♎52'	14°♊52'	Exact
♀ - Qd ☽/♀	12-29-2000	03:19 am	♀ Qd ☽/♀	Ar-Na	23°♑29'	08°♍29'	Exact
♃ -- ☍ ♀	01-01-2001	06:40 pm	♃ ☍ ♀	Tr-Na	02°♊07'℞	02°♐07'	Exact
♅ ---- Qd ☿	01-07-2001	05:05 am	♅ Qd ☿	Tr-Na	18°♒58'	03°♎58'℞	Exact
♇ ---- ☌ Asc	01-09-2001	07:49 pm	♇ ☌ Asc	Tr-Na	14°♐05'	14°♐05'	Exact

♀ = ♃ ★

♃ = ♄

♇ = ♂/M

♇☌A END

"Ian" Time Flow (Cont'd)

General Astrological Considerations about Relationship Difficulty

Perhaps the most common explanations of relationship break-up are the following: *"We outgrew each other; we can't communicate; the relationship changed somehow; I simply cannot stand my partner's craziness."*

These reasons suggest individual development *away from* the original growth path of the relationship. Marriage always begins with big plans for where it will grow; it is a major promotion of a new way and level of life for both partners. When one of the partners takes on highly individualized growth dynamics, when his or her individuality becomes more emphasized than the relationship will easily tolerate, the union begins to break up; a "craziness" has begun.

Uranus

For example, the planet Uranus is traditionally the signal of disruption, often sudden, always definitive. When Uranus by Arc or transit conjoins or squares an Angle (or the Sun; *the significator of the 7th ; or the Sun/Moon midpoint*), there is a signal for change, for intensification of the individual: with the Midheaven, the focus is intensely on the job and/or social status, a new home; with the Ascendant, personal growth including very often the dimension of relocation, starting over again, "up a notch" somewhere else. Note that the Uranus contact with the Ascendant is an opposition to the Descendant: the *individual* dynamic works against the relationship harmony, the relationship routine.[46]

At Uranian times, the balance of individuation within relationship must be inspected. Again, it is expected in our society that the man leads the way in such change and development; the wife is supposed to hold things together

---

46 Naturally, when these measurements—the Arcs and Transits of the outer planets—occur in the horoscope at a very young age, when the child is still at home under the aegis of the parents, the suggested corresponding manifestations are through the parents.

and go along with the man. But what if it is the *woman's* Angles (or Sun) that are being charged with a Uranus Arc or Transit?

If the woman is not able in her reality (not employed, staying at home) to express this Uranian happening reasonably at her social position, *her horoscope can be analyzed for her husband* by seeing her fourth cusp derivatively as her husband's Midheaven (the tenth of the 7th), her Ascendant as *his* contact with the public, her Midheaven as *his* fourth. This derivative House reading is very efficient when the relationship is in healthy balance. When there is difficulty in the relationship, the individual emphasis in development will be disruptive.[47]

The Uranus hard aspect with the Sun is a call to independence, e.g., starting one's own business, and this independence can easily jar, strain, or threaten the relationship.

Neptune

At Neptunian times—when Arcing or Transiting Neptune contacts the Angles or Sun or Moon by conjunction square or opposition, or the significator of the 7th or the Sun/Moon midpoint—the individual within the relationship will probably suffer a suppression of self, a period of lone introspection, even depression. This is tantamount to ego wipe-out and, as such, imbalances the relationship. The reasons/causes are usually vague, intangible, confusing, but the bewilderment is all too real, and so is the demand upon the partner to explore the grace of intimacy and be supportive, rather than blaming, criticizing, rejecting.

Saturn

Saturn times for an individual correspond to intense developmental focus on ambition. Perhaps developments bring the sense of "down times," of hard work for little immediate reward. This can introduce fatigue, dullness, even

---

47 For explanation of Derivative House Readings, please see *Synthesis & Counseling in Astrology*, beginning p. 268.

fear and a sense of futility into the relationship, and the burdens of such concerns tax relationship and usually drain off any sexual bonding energy. Intimacy is the window for support and understanding, but if intimacy is fragile at best, the drain on the relationship in Saturn times can be considerable. A disruption of the relationship may be scapegoat for the anxieties being absorbed from elsewhere; someone/something has to be blamed.

Pluto

Pluto times are very strong times for personal change. Life perspective is usually altered, and this corresponds often with a power struggle, a decision stand-off in relationship *unless* intimacy allows unafraid, real communication and decision-making between the two in relationship. A very important signal is the transit of Pluto square its natal position and, of course, in connection with the ruler of the 7th and/or the Sun/Moon midpoint.

Indirect Midpoints

Certain Solar Arc Indirect Midpoint Pictures (Solar Arc aspects to natal midpoints[48]) can also signal a potential demand upon relationship, usually of less duration (perhaps one or two months) than Direct Arcs or outer planet transits:

- Any outer planet (or SA Mars) fourth harmonic contact with Sun/Moon (relationship archetype).
- Outer planet contact with Sun/Venus (compromising the affections).
- Outer planet contact with Sun/Uranus (issues of independence).
- Uranus or Node=Sun/Neptune (relationship disputes, deception).
- Saturn=Sun/Pluto (power struggle, ruthlessness).
- Neptune=Sun/Node (feeling that relationships are threatening or bothersome; feeling let down by others).

---

48 Please see *Solar Arcs,* which includes an appendix of over 1,000 Indirect Midpoint Pictures.

- Pluto=Sun/MC (changes in life perspective; upset in relationships).
- Asc=Moon/Neptune (feeling a loss of ego definition).
- Pluto=Saturn/Neptune (strong depression; feeling downtrodden; fear).

Indeed there are many more Indirect Midpoint Pictures that can introduce the consideration of tension in relationship, e.g., Uranus=Saturn/MC, "a great new effort, intensity, a new way of doing things, sudden job crisis or family upset"; Uranus=Jupiter/Saturn, "terrible upset with the status of things, forceful change of direction," but these listed here are most important and readily understandable. Such developments threaten to upset many dimensions of life, unless the intimacy, the *rapport*, in the relationship allows growth, change, and vision.

Time-Flow

In the time-flow of relationship over the years, there will be many times of testing signaled by Arcs and Transits as outlined above. Strong contact with the Sun/Moon midpoint is extremely sensitive; strong contact with the significator of the 7th (usually the ruler of the seventh cusp) should not be overlooked. We can test these times in the pas*t to learn of the reaction profile of the partners*. A clear pattern quickly emerges, and, should developmental tension be raising itself as an issue now or in the near future, the reaction profile will undoubtedly be echoed yet again.

The Way of Relationship Counsel

In our work with our clients, we become partners in their process of becoming. With study and experience, we learn to go deeply into understanding the dimensions of individuation: the potentials, the filters and pressures, the frustrations and rewards, *and* the enormous challenges of relationship. In their respect for our skill and sensitivity, our clients expect us to counsel and advise them with wisdom and strategy, often in situations of great complexity. We have to know what we can do and how far we can go.

While most of us are not psychologist, sexologist, *and marriage counselor,* we are expected to know the lay of the land (and the heavens) in these areas, more than just superficially. We are expected to provide insight into these and other areas of life development. As we serve our clients, we build our reputations on the tenor and expertise of our consultations.

Astrology is our system of guidelines. It mirrors a person's development within time. The astrologer's information and insight are channeled *through the astrological networks of symbols* ***into the reality being lived by the client, its past, its present, and its projected future.*** How full we must be to presume to be helpful to others.

This concluding section of our study of intimacy, sexuality, and relationships is devoted to the humanistic and astrological considerations that *can* help us with counsel in relationship difficulty. These considerations are framed within the complex developmental interplay among societal role expectations for male and female, the influence and model of our parents, the fulfillment/frustration balance of our individual needs in relation to environmental prescriptions, and the idealistic projections—the bubbles—we place upon the relationships we make.

Explaining Intimacy

We astrologers should have a well-practiced explanation of intimacy—that state of poise and confidence within ourselves that allows self-presentation to another *with minimal fear of criticism, rejection, and abandonment.* It is never too late for a person to develop into, toward that self-respecting, confident state.

This is vitally important for the client who is approaching a marriage or desperately seeking relationship, or for a tired partner who needs to take stock anew. Often, one person's poise will in turn present an example for the other, for emulation; "ground rules" for interaction are easier to set; the strength of realism displaces idealistic projections.

Throughout the consultation, to help the clients build toward intimacy, we should explain what their parents expected of them; what they needed and still need for themselves; what they have carried forward from those tense developmental times in terms of their self-worth profile, their ability to give love and to receive it, their feeling of not being lovable, should that be the case, and how that has conditioned their relationship history.

It is so difficult to disclose the self, to open up and share, free of the fears of criticism, rejection, and abandonment, when one was unable to do so with the parents in the early homelife. Seeing this, understanding it—how one can be caught in the parents' traffic pattern and completely lost in the hubbub—*can start the rebuilding phase of self-development.*

It is objectivity and understanding of individual life development that allow intimacy to develop as the grace that facilitates mature relationship. The more we know and understand, the less we fear being "found out," as it were, having our vulnerabilities discovered and criticized, being rejected and eventually abandoned. We should illustrate the idealistic bubble-images we create to justify relationships, how they burst and how poor behaviors emerge. We should dramatize the concept of being real and practical within the beginnings of love and within the maintenance of love.

It is sometimes revelatory to point out to a client that the defenses we build for ourselves in early development are *not needed so urgently, so continuously as we get older*, that we have literally outgrown many of the problematic concerns and situations that haunted early development. Those defenses are simply **routines we have never abandoned** and they use up a great deal of energy that could be applied afresh into new directions of growth. They confine. They restrict growth. They *can* be relaxed, along with the off-putting behaviors that accompany them. Have we taken stock of ourselves lately to see *how well developed we are in spite of all that has gone on before?* What can be shared with the clients to help them delight in themselves? *What can we point out to clients to have them like themselves sincerely, better than ever before?*

What are the fine, admirable points *about the partner*? How has he or she grown—improved—over time since the beginning of the relationship? What difficulties have been overcome? How did one partner help the other? How do those attributes and cooperation work together to help the relationship grow more? *Building these positive support concepts is most welcomed by the client in trouble. The client can leave the consultation feeling better, stronger, fortified.*

Our explanation about intimacy need not be a long lecture. Since the pressure within the mandate to relate is so great, the client will quickly understand the fear he or she has about exposing personal vulnerabilities, about criticism, rejection, and abandonment. The client will appreciate how understanding development and discarding old routines of thought and behavior can bring fresh poise and confidence. The poise against criticisms, rejection, and abandonment through inner knowledge and strength should flavor the entire remedial section of the consultation.

Capsulating the Shortcomings

The astrologer has tracked the client's development astrologically to the present. The discussion of that development has disclosed the reality profile of difficulties, significances, defenses, and routines of reaction. Together, the client and astrologer can capsulate the personal shortcomings that have been brought forward in time and inhibited the most fulfilling development.[49]

The point is that we creatively summarize the developmental concerns objectively. *That objectivity is freeing*; sometimes the change of mood, thought, and behavior occurs quite quickly; almost always, a new feel is given to development especially in the relationship. Figuratively, the behavioral/attitudinal constructs that have proved problematic can be "put into a box and placed up there on a shelf," out of the mind's way. A knowing separation must take place between the past and the now with regard to the problems. There are better things to think about to empower further growth. Not much can be done about those past situations except *to separate from them and change the value judgments we have given them during development.*

---

49 The capsulations can take the form of the short profiling that summarizes (introduce) many of the cases used in this book, without the astrological jargon, of course.

Conflicts and Anger

Conflict is always part of the growth process. Muscles grow in strength through resistance to contrary forces; people grow through the interaction and the struggle between the need pressures of the inner environment and the prescriptions of the outer environment; relationships grow through the interaction of two individuals exploring shared strengths and compromise to help the relationship grow fulfillingly for the family.

The vitality and necessity of conflicts—developmental tension—are seen in the horoscope hologram through the Angular, Succedent, and Cadent Crosses of Houses.[50] Each cross contains zones of developmental experience in unalterable square relationship to each other; the interplay of concerns within each Cross are essential to growth. There *must* be tension—with parents, for example—because *it is through our management of the tension and our assimilation of the learning within the process that we define who we become*—our Ascendant projection on the cross axis to the parental axis, into relationships and the public in the 7th.

In life and in astrology, growth is not a concern of whether there was tension or not, but, rather, *how much tension* was there and *how was it assimilated* into life development.

How do we manage conflict when it occurs? Do we manage it as we saw our parents manage it? A recent client has Mars at her seventh cusp quindecile Pluto, ruler of her 5th (children, giving love): her whole life has been self-isolating (within a Grand Trine) for protection from early homelife neglect, and the behaviors she modeled in this process are now evidenced in her daughter; the mother says "She is just like me, but four times worse, and we do not speak." The problems with the child, now an adult, obsess my client; *they are a displacement of her own.*

Anger is a vitally important defense reaction. It is with us at birth; it is natural; tests have shown that anger emerges in babies at the six-month age

---

50 Please see Tyl, *Synthesis & Counseling in Astrology*, 225–270.

period, just before fears develop. Aggression forms to express anger and force gratification to occur.[51]

Astrologically, we know that Mars in the 12th, especially within 10 or 12 degrees of the Ascendant corresponds with anger that is hidden away in the personality, often eating away at structures working for need fulfillment. Some frustration and upset have been internalized (usually at the age of the Arc measure Mars=Ascendant) dysfunctionally.

How does the client manage anger within conflict? Is there respect for the partner's position, or is blame the chief reaction? Is an established intimacy allowing anger to be expressed reasonably, constructively?

We will often hear from a male client under relationship pressure, "She tells me I'm *always* letting her down." A statement like this is extremely debilitating. The operable word here, "always," is irrational (and probably a negative animus projection by the wife): he is *not* letting her down *always*; this is something that cannot be substantiated, but the statement of the extreme is final and permanent; there is no answer to it except, "No, I do not," and this goes nowhere.[52]

Perhaps he is letting her down, in her perception, something like 43 percent of the time, or 72 percent! Using these terms to clarify the complaint actually can introduce healing humor to defuse the rigid, vengeful accusation and allow a respectful discussion to begin. The objective of course is for the angry partners within a conflict to submit to each other a list, to *communicate what needs are not being fulfilled*; then, something *can* be done about the problem if both partners stay poised and avoid brick-wall criticisms and rejection within the discussion.

There can be change for the good for one partner that threatens the other, if intimacy, working together, is not active in the relationship. The husband

---

51 Tyl, *Synthesis & Counseling in Astrology*, 725–729.

52 Extremism like this falls into the fallacy of dichotomous reasoning: it is untenable to portray an emotionally perceived situation in absolute terms of positive or negative. There are many shades, degrees in between.

getting a major job promotion and possibly a relocation assignment can threaten the family with insecurity, leaving the established relationships in the community, the children's school; the wife feels threatened with being "left behind" in many ways (especially, say, if her Moon is in Taurus, a resistance to change for fear of transient insecurity).

The wife returning to the work place will tax her energies and time greatly and take attention away from the family unit and the husband in particular. The husband can suffer jealousy, even feel competition from the wife. The situation threatens to expose his vulnerabilities. Doesn't he earn enough money? Are the wife's personal needs being overlooked? Is he to blame?

Occurrences like these—events of any kind, really—have no value *until we give them value*. What value will the wife give her husband's promotion, what value will the husband give his wife's plan for individual growth? It is along these lines that the client should be encouraged to pursue the fulfilling resolution of conflict. Assessment of value to any event is of enormous importance with regard to how functionally or dysfunctionally the event is fitted into the scheme of life.

A thirty-two-year-old client, "Beth," lives with a man in a good relationship. From a previous marriage, he has a son who is often with him and his girlfriend in their home. Beth now desperately wants to have a child of her own with this man; he is reluctant because he feels the child, another child, will complicate his business growth and relocation plans, etc. This is a conflict that grows deeply between them as each month goes on; Beth feels that time is running out for her.

Beth tends to be strong with words (Mercury in Capricorn squared by Jupiter) and explosive with temperament (peregrine Mars in the 12th). Her first instinct was to just stop taking her contraceptive pill. Of course, this is dishonest within the relationship and would taint the child, perhaps for a lifetime; it would introduce distrust between Beth and her man that would probably never end.

The objective became to set a respectable time limit for the man to think things through; avoid the introduction of anger and frustration into hot argument; and preserve Beth's integrity within her natural, intense desire to fulfill herself by birthing a child (Moon-Venus in Aquarius quindecile the Midheaven; $Pluto_{Asc}$ sextile Neptune5).

Explaining this to Beth *calmed her down*; the appreciation of the situation objectively gave her some distance, and she could create a plan of communication to her boyfriend.

The consultation took place in March 2001. *SA Neptune, ruler of her 5th, would conjoin her Sun in February 2002, with SP Moon simultaneously squaring her Midheaven*. This was clearly a time that could correspond to having a baby, nine–ten months from the consultation date, or it could be a time of tremendous bewilderment, a confused evaluation and breakdown of her love relationship with her boyfriend. In every way, in the expanded present of the consultation, it was grow-up time.

We determined that she would write a rational, keenly expressive letter to her boyfriend, edit it carefully, keeping it as short as possible. The letter set a target date of January 1, 2002, for his decision to be with her in this life-dream of hers to have a child. The letter made it very clear as well that she would be "*with him* all the way" in his work plans, including a far-reaching relocation.

The clincher on this plan for Beth was my suggestion that this conflict, being managed with grace now, *would establish a clear evaluation of her relationship and its future soon, within nine months*. The clarity of all this promised her a resolution that would affect much of her life to come; while that was portentous, it would be definite, clear, and secure. And much of the conflict was defused.

Many clients need help with communication, especially within angry, conflicting situations, *away from the communication channels routined over many years with the same person*. But the objective must remain dominatingly clear:

personal growth in respectful relation to another within the goals set for the relationship itself.

Psychiatrist David Viscott writes: "Sometimes a relationship does break apart when one partner changes. The surest way to destroy a relationship is for one partner to stand in the way of the other partner's self-fulfillment. If you think about it, that goes against everything a relationship stands for. A partner should be able to rely on the other's love and support to help him grow into the person he feels destined to be. To stand in the way is the same thing as saying, I don't want you to be yourself."[53]

This does not mean that conflict is resolved by capitulation, giving in to the partner's every whim. It means that listening, empathizing, and respecting are the keys to progress in compromise, in intimate togetherness, and that may indeed involve seeing the light in terms of capitulation, with both persons being fulfilled by it. Gone must be the destroyers: criticism, rejection, and the threat of abandonment.

Psychotherapist Harriett Lerner observes: "Intimacy means that we can be who we are in a relationship, and allow the other person to do the same . . . this means we can stay emotionally connected to that other party who thinks, feels, and believes differently, without needing to change, convince, or fix the other."[54]

Within our society's view of managing conflict, the prescription that the woman should sacrifice her "I" for the "we" of the relationship led by the man is very strong. The woman under tension, expected to be the one who keeps the family together, suffers terribly from her threatened loss of identity. The male should know this; and empathy with the woman should season the discussion to resolve conflict.

Other approaches to conflict resolution that can be recommended by the astrologer are for the two people to write their feelings down respectfully and

53 Viscott, 124.

54 Lerner, *The Dance of Intimacy*, 7.

exchange letters with each other—similar to the technique adopted for Beth (above). Writing a letter about personal needs within a conflict situation and then editing it very carefully *allow temperament and anger to leave the body* and then the message can be shared reasonably or even discarded and not presented at all. The letter allows a real measurement of objectification: the feelings are "out there," and a reply can be carefully prepared, or the catharsis of writing then is complete, and the issue evaporates or solves itself.[55]

Discussions can be held on the telephone at a planned time: there is a give-and-take behavioral protocol well established for telephone conversations that helps to keep order in the discussion of conflict.

When one is traveling far from home, one is usually more oneself than when at home under the prescriptions of the relationship. From that different perspective, discussion can often be pursued more honestly and more courteously; the two persons are not threatening each other by their presence.

It is extremely important that no conflict discussion take place in the dark, in bed, for example: faces cannot be seen to register emotional coloring of statements. Additionally, arguing in bed, the usual setting for love-making, taints the scene with discord.

Sexuality

It is lovely—and indeed intimate—to ponder that, when a relationship is right, people make love in many ways all the time.

Viscott says, "Making love is to do something kind for the other person. Making love means that you not only care for the other person's feelings as your own but that you act on your caring to make him/her aware of your love. Making love is the ultimate in thoughtfulness, in considering the other person's feelings."[56]

---

55 How often have you written an intensely angry note/letter to someone and then realized that the anger had been discharged in the process, and that it was no longer necessary or advisable to send the letter off?

56 Viscott, 113.

Most people seem not to have thought about this, since they are so tied up with sexual performance, with meeting a Hollywood/*Playboy*/*Cosmopolitan*, even pornographic standard. Indeed sexuality *is* vitally a part of who we are and what we share to fulfill relationship, but its complications—so inextricably involved as sexuality is with individual needs, self-image, prescriptions of society, and the modeling by the parents—its complications easily cloud the joys, and impersonality all too often displaces empathy in the union.

When a sexual problem exists between two people, it most often suggests, reflects a problem in their *relationship*, not necessarily a specific problem with sexuality. That problem may then be exacerbated by a lack of sex information [poor communication] and poor sex technique [bumbling involvement, selfish perspective]. As we have seen, difficulties usually stem from early developmental conditioning: suppression, guilt, fears, bad relationship history, trauma, in relation to the individual's needs for sexual expression, but the core of the problem originates within the *rapport* between the two persons in the relationship, within how they relate to each other *in other matters*. When the difficulty manifests in the sexual life, the problem has gone a long way in its development.

For example, if a man or woman has shown him- or herself to be less than the original idealized projection—when a bubble has burst—sensual attraction between them drops dramatically. Sexual performance frequency drops off. Performance itself becomes routined, selfish, and it is focused on tranquilization rather than emotional fulfillment. The sensual is dehumanized. Boredom gives way to rejection. The first step is a tacit agreement to no sex, then to separate bedrooms. And it is extraordinary how children, even at age six or seven, and certainly older, become awkwardly and sadly aware of this spectrum of tensions between their parents. The modeling image for the children is deeply marred.

At the same time, it must be recognized that superb sexual harmony between two people can offset deficiencies each has with the other *elsewhere in the relationship*. The partners will look to the sexual union as a way, as their best way, to confirm the relationship. But as well, this eventually brings difficulty as time and age change hormone production, body form, and mindset and sexuality loses its top hierarchical need position for the couple. Other dimensions within the relationship must move up the ladder in importance for the growth of the union to continue, and if these dimensions have remained flawed in the partners' individual perspectives, the relationship will develop critical problems. Sexuality can no longer be the solve-all dimension of the union.

Communication about sexuality is a very important activity that can put problems into the light of discussion and resolution, i.e., the problems one person may feel about the other can be discussed as they begin to invade the sexual area of experience. The male needs the female's "assessment" of his sexual ability, and open communication about this, with grace and mutual exploration, can benefit both male *and* female. This evaluation *stands for an evaluation of the male in other dimensions of the relationship* and, as such, it is very far-reaching.

The female needs to know that she is exciting to the male, that she is alluring, and open communication about this, with grace and innovation, can benefit both. Problems in other areas of the relationship may be threatening to intrude on the sexual area of experience—her gaining weight, for example—and good communication can open up a shared responsibility for this, and understanding of how to solve the problem together.

At the same time, with good communication about sexuality, each partner can share what is important for sexual fulfillment, which can range from a particular erogenous zone or technique to enactment of very private fantasy. The point is that the two persons are brought closer and closer together, one helping the other to fulfillment, *as one helps the other into directions of growth through other areas of life experience.*

Again, intimacy is the key to the harmony that allows a fine sexual relationship, i.e., a relationship that fulfills individual needs, mindset, and fantasies, all in the embrace of sharing emotional care and support.

Interestingly, fidelity in our times now is not the stringent issue it used to be. Statistics show that 50–60 percent of men are unfaithful in their marriage and between 40 and 45 percent among the women. It is clear that fidelity is a demand half the people cannot meet. But research further shows that most affairs are casual, not involving deep commitments; they arise out of boredom or from the need for excitement, as a convenience, as an effort to make up for something missing in the life, or in the interest of discovering another human being in a speeded-up intimacy process that overlooks the shortcomings that perhaps are reiterated daily in criticisms in the marriage.

Sexuality is rarely the issue that breaks up marriages. **A lack of understanding, the need to share something special**—those are the driving forces for separation. When the discovery of infidelity initially enflames someone to blinding hurt and anger, one runs the risk of missing the point: *the sexual activity is a symptom of other problems.*

On this subject, Viscott suggests that "If you hurt your partner by such an act [sexual dalliance], it is very likely an act of anger [Mars: sex, anger]. People who get involved sexually and end up hurting their partner are often simply angry people using the most painful weapon they know even if they protest that they had no control over the situation. . . . A sexual encounter used in this way can be one of the cruelest things you can do, for it not only says 'I am angry' but also 'You are worthless.' "[15]

Ideally, sexual fidelity in a relationship should develop not by prescription but by choice.

We can see easily how these thoughts can be introduced into the consultation when called for, when the client discloses that criticisms in the marriage are focused, in displacement, upon sexual performance or the lack of it.

It is extremely important with this very sensitive issue that, in the consultation, the astrologer put aside *personal* opinions/preferences about sexuality. The astrologer may have a terribly complex and/or frustrated sex life, an

---

15 Viscott, 77.

Olympic need and capacity for sexual expression, or a difficulty with intimacy in her or his relationship, but *the dedication to what is possible for fulfillment in the client's reality is of paramount importance in the consultation*. The astrologer's value judgments based upon defense of the personal position play no role, and very often, in sharing knowledge, in teaching with a client, the astrologer's personal concerns are themselves objectified and energies are freed.

And we astrologers must know how far we can go within our discipline. Sexual difficulties brought forward from *critical* events, abuse trauma, enormous disillusionment about the parents early in development often require extended specialist attention, and the astrologer should be ready with referrals and the way to arrange for the client *finally* to get assistance with the problem.

One female client spoke most openly about her lifelong block with sexual orgasm. A marriage had broken up, with this problem a central pivot-point symptom. In my work with her in astrological consultation, I spotted a period of three years, when she was thirteen to sixteen, in which she simply could not remember anything (and it was astrologically highly charged). She was intrigued with the possibility of selective amnesia; I urged her to visit a hypnotist, on my referral. I told the hypnotist of my finding; the hypnotist was able to unlock those years from her memory and cause her to bring them forward into conscious discussion. A schoolteacher had sexually molested her. Now that that was known, the situation could be objectified through analysis and the emotionality of it defused. The therapy led to freedom of sexual response.

A sixty-two-year-old male client had hidden his failing erectile capacity from his wife for several years (in the confidentiality of the consultation, he was relieved to share the secret with me); sex between them had ceased. His wife (also a client) simply had taken the situation in stride (the tolerance and self-sacrifice expected of a woman according to societal prescription) and, to satisfy her strong sexuality profile, kept sexually active through masturbation. I actually phoned my referent urologist, during the consultation with the husband, to make the appointment for the man—and the urologist was able to alleviate the problem and get the man back on track. Then we worked on other issues within the relationship to regain the intimacy that had flourished before. The man simply had been too embarrassed to seek help, and it was the authority of my referral that somehow broke the ice.

In the consultation, I believe the creative astrologer can be most helpful by making creative connections throughout the client's development history, with particular reference to the themes covered in this book, guided by the appropriate astrology, to bring those creative connections together in a developmental scenario that reveals the client's need profile, value judgments, and relationship history (parents, schooling, relationships, job structures, family, etc.).

The astrologer is keenly aware of cycle and can relate past measurements and developments to measurements and plans for the future.

The greatest therapeutic service is to suggest an understanding of events in development in order to free up rigid defense routines. This will help to diminish routined fears, build self-appreciation, and establish the poise that makes intimacy and mature relationship possible.

A New Agreement

Wedding days are major celebrations: two people have finally "found each other," *one of their major life tasks has been achieved.* The ceremonial vows include reference to permanence, "for better or for worse, in sickness and in health, until death do you part." This is a serious acknowledgement that there will be difficulty in the marriage: conflicts between the people, battles with the environment that drain off energy from each other, turns of fate, burst bubbles, BUT the union *shall prevail* and actually help set things straight once again. The vows often include the subject of (sexual) faithfulness, introducing a tremendous specter of tension, guilt, devisiveness, and shame into the prospects of the union, especially for the couple who are young and unexposed to so much of life.

The individuals in the marriage *do* have troubles with the tensions required for growth. The idealized projections one makes to the other break up; negative animus and anima behaviors signal the burst bubbles. Criticisms lead to rejection, and rejection can lead to abandonment. What can restore the poise of intimacy? What information holds things together?

Note the observation about the marriage that so often accompanies trauma—like the perilous sickness or death of a child or one of the partners, a natural disaster or a terrible accident, or even discovered adultery: the partners say, "This has been difficult, but it has brought us closer together," or, "This has strengthened our marriage." There has been a wake-up call—a reality blow—that has revealed the humanness of the partners and their need for the support of each other.

It is so very easy for partners to lose their organization of values: caught up in the swirl of individual need fulfillment (on the job, the lure of advancement and change, for example), each can lose reference to support for the other and to where the relationship itself is going. It is exceedingly difficult to make the right choices in relationship when one is still searching for who one is individually. It is immaturity that stimulates idealistic projections and wish fulfillment substituting for realism.

A formalized Renewed Agreement is very helpful to stabilize things. The couple can work out independently and then together a renewed marriage agreement that recognizes their maturing capabilities, their uncovered needs, and their developing dreams. This can be ceremonially celebrated, much as some couples actually redo the wedding ceremony (usually with the original vows).

The point here is that, with a formalized, Renewed Agreement, *more realistic promises are used*, which bring the individuals more practicably together; there will be fewer compulsions to criticize or to reject each other; there will be renewed accord. And there will be new commitment.

In a much less compelling sense, this is what is expected to happen when people take a strategic trip away from tension, "leaving the scene of difficulty,"

difficulty should vanish. The long weekend trip or, indeed, relocation does not do the job of restoration since *one takes oneself along wherever one goes*. The problem is within the developmental matrix of the relationship, not exclusively at the scene of the relationship or in its timeframe, as we have seen repeatedly in our study.

A Renewed Agreement often *can* work to stabilize things. Specific dimensions are brought out of the individual and put down on paper. Communication in this way can be edited objectively, nonthreateningly. Finally, the finished product has the imprimatur of both persons, and there is improved harmony.

These are thoughts about the way of relationship counsel that I think are accessible to the nonspecialist astrologer and acceptable by the client within the frame of the astrological consultation. They issue informed and practical out of astrological measurements of individual needs, developmental interaction in the early home, giving and receiving love, level of education, communication facility, and relationship history.

Considering the weave of intimacy, love, romance, and sexuality as we have studied these subjects *brings our horoscope to a different level of potential helpfulness in matters of relationship*. This applies to homosexual as well as to heterosexual relationships: relationships are relationships, two people trying to living together for the improvement of their lives.

Often in our studies here, we have read the benefits of astrological counsel *in the words of clients who have had the experience*. They have learned to understand their growth, the problems they are managing, and how the process has helped them mature in life with others. Astrology is an extraordinary mirror of life development, and the astrologer is a vitally important, reactive witness to the reflections.

It is important to note that very much of our study has necessarily had a strong orientation to the woman. This reflects the societal prescription that it is women who hold relationships together, that they are the ones who are *supposed to.* It is relatively infrequent that a man comes to an astrologer to understand relationship problems, to keep a relationship together.

Regardless of what our society expects for relationships, living happily ever after is difficult. But the effort to do so—to grow, to mature, to reach the sun—challenges individuality into being, as much as it creates the relationships that are necessary for humanity to continue, as we propagate after our kind.

Bibliography

Bold-face titles mark books of exceptional readability and special value to the issues of this volume and its preparation.

Aronson, Elliot. ***The Social Animal.*** New York: Freeman & Co, 1994 (seventh edition).

Banzhaf, Hajo, and Brigitte Theler. *Secrets of Love & Partnership.* York Beach, Maine: Samuel Weiser, 1998.

Gray, John. ***Men Are from Mars, Women Are from Venus.*** New York: HarperCollins, 1992.

Green, Jeffrey. *Pluto—Volume II.* St. Paul: Llewellyn Publications, 1997.

Lerner, Harriet. ***The Dance of Anger.*** New York Harper Perennial, 1986.

____. ***The Dance of Intimacy.*** New York: Harper Perennial, 1990.

Moore, Marcia, and Mark Douglas. ***Astrology, The Divine Science.*** York Harbor, Maine: Arcane, 1978.

Moore, Thomas. *Care of the Soul.* New York: Harper Perennial, 1992.

____. *The Soul of Sex.* New York: HarperCollins, 1998.

____. *Soul Mates.* New York: HarperCollins, 1994.

Sanford, John. ***The Invisible Partners.*** New York: Paulist Press, 1980.

Sullivan, Erin. ***Dynasty.*** Arkana-London/New York: Penguin Books, 1996.

Tyl, Noel. *Holistic Astrology: The Analysis of Inner and Outer Environments.* St. Paul: TAI/Llewellyn Publications, 1980.

____. *The Astrological Timing of Critical Illness.* St. Paul: Llewellyn Publications, 1998.

____. ***The Creative Astrologer.*** St. Paul: Llewellyn Publications, 2000.

_____. ***Sexuality in the Horoscope,*** Noel Tyl, ed. St. Paul: Llewellyn Publications, 1994.

_____. ***Synthesis & Counseling in Astrology***. St. Paul: Llewellyn Publications, 1994.

Viscott, David, M.D. ***How to Live with another Person.*** New York: Pocket Books, 1976.

Index

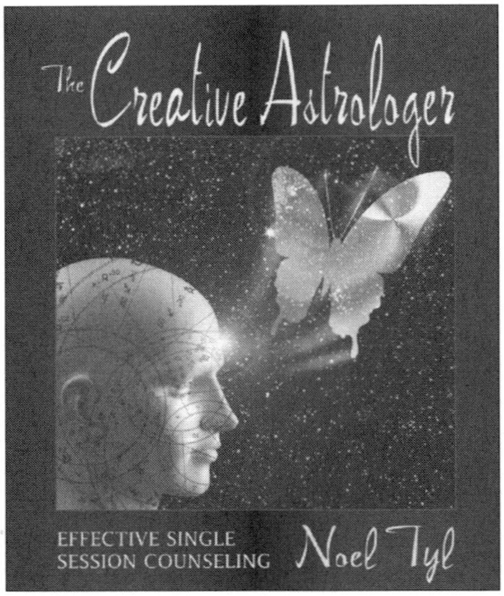

The Creative Astrologer

Effective Single-Session Counseling

Noel Tyl

The Creative Astrologer is a new point of departure for astrology: the realm of counseling effectiveness in a single-session format. For more than thirty years, renowned astrologer Noel Tyl has brought psychological methodology into astrological symbolism and analysis. Now he crowns that effort with a master volume emphasizing the techniques of counseling as part of modern astrological practice.

Tyl offers more than 700 creative connections to guide astrologers throughout planetary and aspect symbolisms into deep analysis of the human condition. He clearly develops the art of questioning, techniques for inviting disclosure, and specific objectification therapies. Every analytical insight comes from his own long career of experience, theorization, and experimentation. Verbatim examples from his own recent client sessions are used to illustrate his techniques.

1-56718-740-4, 264 pp., 7½ x 9⅛ **$17.95**

Astrological Timing of Critical Illness

Early Warning Patterns in the Horoscope

Noel Tyl

Foreword by Mitchell Gibson, M.D.
Introduction by Jeffrey Wolf Green

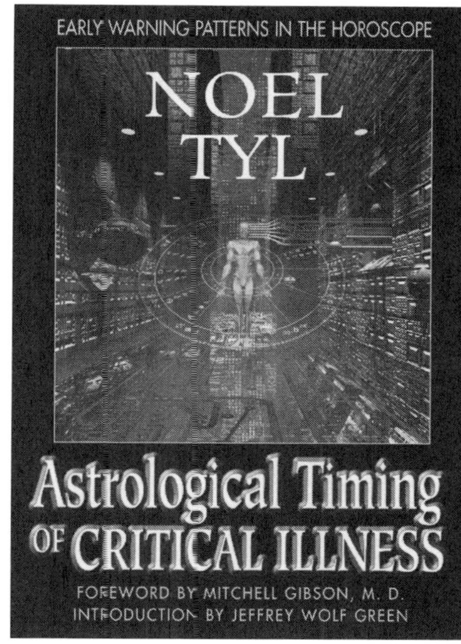

Now, through master astrologer Noel Tyl's work, astrology has a thoroughly tested method with which to understand and anticipate the emergence of critical illness: from the natal horoscope, throughout development, and within the aging process. Astrologers can use Noel Tyl's discovery to work with people to extend life as much as possible, to live a full life, and to do it all with holistic understanding.

Tyl painstakingly researched more than seventy cases to test his patterning discoveries Your analytical skill will be alerted, tested, and sharpened through these very same cases, which include notables such as Carl Sagan (bone cancer), Betty Ford (breast cancer), Larry King (heart attack), Norman Schwarzkopf (prostate cancer), and Mike Wallace (manic depression), and many others.

- Explore the predisposition to pathology as indicated in the horoscope
- Learn the aspect patterns natally that, with Solar Arcs and Transits, reveal extreme challenge to the life system
- Exercise your observational skills and your facility reading planetary networks and timing patterns through the study of 70 horoscopes
- Lead your clients to seek early medical attention that could save lives

1-56718-738-2, 288 pp., 7 x 10, charts **$19.95**

To Order Call 1-800-THE MOON
Prices subject to change without notice